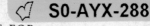
<small>PRAISE FOR</small>
Strong at the Broken Places

"Extraordinary."

—Larry King

"Career journalist Cohen doesn't flinch from probing for truth about relationships, money, fear, and death. . . . One only hopes that, with their group presentation to a class of Harvard medical students, these five taught young medicos as much as they could teach Cohen and through him, us." —*Booklist*

"*Strong at the Broken Places* opens our minds and hearts to the harsh realities experienced by people living every minute with chronic, debilitating illnesses. In sharp detail, these stories express the strength of the human spirit in the face of crushing adversity. They serve as a lesson, teaching us the values of compassion and acceptance, and reminding us that despite any hardship, the soul can prevail." —Rosalynn Carter

"For a long time, my toughest foe was the man standing opposite me on a cream-colored cotton canvas. Today, the fight of my life is with an incurable disease—the toughest of foes. Striking back at illness is a common struggle for millions of us. . . . *Strong at the Broken Places* is a book for America because it tells the real-life stories of real people coping with devastating conditions who fight hard every day. . . . They are the winners." —Muhammad Ali

"The strength of these profiles derives from Cohen's focus on chronic illnesses that, as he notes, are not 'sexy' and generally 'do not resolve themselves.' . . . These are stories dense with quotidian details."

—*Washington Post*

"This unusual book gives a voice to the voiceless—the chronically disabled who, in our health-conscious society, are defined by their disease. . . . In this advocacy book, written like a personal journal, Cohen tells their stories. . . . *Strong at the Broken Places* ends on a note of hope."

—*Providence Journal*

PRAISE FOR
Blindsided

"*Blindsided* is beautifully written and utterly honest. May we all be so brave and caring in our families."

—Tom Brokaw

"Eloquent and brutally honest."

—*Seattle Times*

"*Blindsided* is a powerful memoir, tough in the way Cohen's old news bosses would have wanted to be tough. It doesn't flinch and it doesn't whine."

—*New York Times Book Review*

"A warm, sarcastic, unflinching dissection of love, pain, laughter, and wounded pride."

—*Chicago Tribune*

"A powerful and agonizingly frank description of a life with which many chronically ill people and their families will identify. . . . Highly recommended."

—*Library Journal* (starred review)

About the Author

RICHARD M. COHEN is the author of *Blindsided: Lifting a Life Above Illness*, a *New York Times* bestseller. He is the host of *Strong at the Broken Places*, a broadcast on WABC Radio that examines issues associated with chronic illnesses. For twenty-five years he worked as a network television news producer, winning numerous journalism awards, including three Emmys and a George Foster Peabody. He lives outside New York City with his wife, Meredith Vieira, and their children.

Also by Richard M. Cohen

Blindsided: Lifting a Life Above Illness

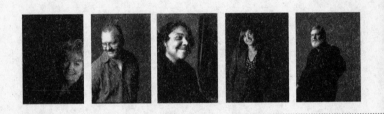

HARPER

NEW YORK • LONDON • TORONTO • SYDNEY

Strong
at the
Broken
Places

*Voices of
Illness, a
Chorus of
Hope*

Richard M. Cohen

Again, for Meredith
and our traveling circus

HARPER

A hardcover edition of this book was published in 2008 by Harper-Collins Publishers.

FIRST HARPER PAPERBACK PUBLISHED 2009.

All photographs by Mark Ostow, © 2008

Designed by Nicola Ferguson

The Library of Congress has catalogued the hardcover edition as follows:
Cohen, Richard M.
    Strong at the broken places: voices of illness, a chorus of hope / Richard M. Cohen. — 1st ed.
        p. cm.
    ISBN 978-0-06-076311-4
1. Chronically ill — United States — Biography. 2. People with disabilities — United States — Biography. I. Title
    RC108.C638 2008
    616'.044—dc22   2007023965

ISBN 978-0-06-076312-1 (pbk.)

09 10 11 12 13 OV/RRD 10 9 8 7 6 5 4 3 2 1

Acknowledgments

THE RIGHT IDEA without any follow-through is dead on arrival. My determination to listen carefully to the voices of the sick, to pry open lives and write the hidden story of illness, begged a practical question. How was I going to find such people?

Admittedly there a certain hubris in thinking that there were suffering people, weary of their own struggles, who would endure yet more probing and agree to share the intimate details of their personal lives. Yet, experience suggested that somewhere in this land were individuals living with serious sickness who knew the frustration of the voice not heard. I would find them, patients who would welcome the opportunity to tell their stories. So many of the sick are lost and want to be found.

Myrl Weinberg and Marc Boutin of the National Health Council in Washington helped identify such people. The NHC is an organization of fifty of the nation's leading patient groups, representing approximately one hundred million people who deal with chronic diseases. They believe in restoring the silenced voice of the guy in the next hospital bed. These good people helped to assemble the cast.

Linda Loewenthal, my literary agent, helped birth this book, sticking around to help raise the difficult child. Anastasia Toufexis, my trusty, unflappable freelance friend, edited, cutting through the underbrush of my prose, which often required a machete.

Gail Winston, an executive editor at HarperCollins, once again gave guidance and, as always, stood by the book. And two others deserve mention for showing up when the going got tough.

Martha Crowninshield, close friend and colleague on the Council of the Harvard NeuroDiscovery Center, believed in this project and was always there in support, leading the charge to make our medical school seminar a reality. Bradie Metheny, a master of matters medical and a patient advocate, shared his knowledge and considerable wisdom with grace. My gratitude goes to the people of Harvard Medical School who offered support and opened their door to a band of patients and a writer on a mission to give voice to the sick.

As always, there is Meredith, who rises at three on most mornings to survey the news she will report. As I worked on this second book, a screaming alarm clock and lights would jar me out of bed and to the computer a little earlier than I wanted. And there I would park. My wife and the crowd of adolescents who hang at our house mostly ignored me. They walked by, sometimes just rolling their eyes. The silent "Oh, please, not again" could only be inferred.

Yes, again, and because of all of you.

The world breaks every one
and afterward many are strong
at the broken places.

—ERNEST HEMINGWAY,
A Farewell to Arms

Contents

Preface

THESE ARE FACES of illness in America. Do not look away. The characters may surprise you, even shatter a stereotype or two. They are people, not cases, survivors, not victims. Quite simply, they are us. They carry shared resolve, a determination to survive. To flourish.

Too often the sick are seen and not heard. Listen. Their songs are soft but steady. Hear the sound of steel, the quiet toughness at the core. Pay attention. These people sing to themselves and, if we choose to listen, to us all. I, too, know sickness and have joined the chorus. We walk together as one, each with an individual identity and unique story.

My story of coping with multiple sclerosis and colon cancer was told in *Blindsided*. That struggle did not end. The book came and went, and a weakening body took no notice. Illness kept cutting its swath. I am angry and hurting, and each day I need to relearn the lessons I had the temerity to believe I could teach. Arms and hands weaken, legs and feet falter. My vision suffers, squints revealing progressively less at any distance. Now I look to others to find the road out of the dark forest.

We, the injured, are everywhere. We are fast becoming a nation of the sick. The numbers do not lie. Chronic illness has become the silent flood, flowing slowly, steadily under our doors. We tumble in slow-motion from safe ground, twisting and struggling to survive in a cold sea of all that we once were and can be no more.

Chronic conditions attack body and spirit, assaulting the quality of our lives. Some are life-threatening. All are life-altering. Ever so slowly, moment by moment, function and sensation cease. Muscles and nerves malfunction. The body's processes grow difficult. Our view of ourselves as normal human beings making our way in a neutral world is challenged as, in the eyes of others, we become our illnesses.

Chronic conditions do not resolve themselves. Unlike terminal illnesses, there is no high drama with these diseases. They are not sexy, and are little noticed or understood by an unknowing public that would prefer not to think about them. Those who are hit hard know the frustration of being marginalized, reduced, and pushed to the side by these chilly attitudes. We are handed a cocktail of condescension and a basket of doubts about our limitations. The crisis of confidence that follows can be contagious, and soon affects every part of our being.

With chronic illness, every facet of a once-robust life is overtaken and redefined. From the ability to find and hold jobs to the capacity to build and sustain personal relationships, the facts of a sick person's world change dramatically. The slow slide down carries us, and we lose control.

Still, we go on. We double the effort, for what is the

option? Too often, we remain silent. We are a hidden population, invisible except to ourselves and those who love us. When I wrote *Blindsided*, I felt alienated and isolated. I now know I am not alone. Many travel the same road, and common ground lies beneath our feet.

We have so much at stake and so much to say, but it can take years of battle with our own demons to recognize the power of what we have to offer one another. Nobody will speak for us with the authority we bring to our own stories. Where so many among us find the resolve and the inner strength to rise up and keep going is a mystery to me. That we do serves as pure inspiration.

This book profiles five strong people on the front lines of illness. Each fights a different war. All are ready to share. Sometimes they hobble, even stumble, but they are extraordinary for their resolve. They will finish on their own steam according to their own terms. They, and their families, speak from the heart and tell their stories with pride.

This gang of five is not timid or shy or self-conscious about their physical flaws. They are unapologetic about their bodies' weaknesses. They try so hard, struggling to travel well on one of life's toughest journeys.

Hemingway had it right. If the world is not the enemy, neither is it our friend. In the end, no matter who surrounds us, we travel alone. Our friends and loved ones are there, providing an infrastructure of love and support. But courage must be drawn from within. Let the world see us as we see ourselves and have the faith to permit us do it our way.

I have been in these people's faces for years, brazen

enough to ask the questions others would be too polite to touch. That was allowed, and so far, we are still talking.

I admire each of these people and am proud to call them my friends.

Richard M. Cohen
June 2007
New York

....

one

The Meeting

MAGICALLY, THE FACES from my book showed themselves as the appointed hour passed. The clocks with their muted chimes tinkled softly, almost mysteriously, from various positions around the old place. Characters were stepping out of the manuscript, a work in progress, to finish the job.

The invited guests, who were meeting for the first time, seemed serious but not at all somber. All were on their best behavior, a bit nervous and looking hard into one another's eyes. They seemed to be searching for something only they could identify.

I had embarked on a journey to see chronic illness through lenses other than my own. I had searched hard for and found a cast of five. For two years, I crisscrossed the country, passing through airports and down highways, listening, probing, and forming a new community with these amazing people.

Slowly, we began to share our troubled lives, our recipes for coping. At hospitals and in homes, on living room couches and at dining room tables, these extraordinary people began to reveal themselves. I heard their stories of sickness and listened hard as they described how their lives were changing.

My journey began on the California coast, northwest of Los Angeles. At the base of the Santa Monica Mountains, I met up with Denise. ALS, a hideous neurodegenerative disease, has redefined life for this woman. No doctor is going to save her. Denise fights to move forward. By choice, she stands alone. "Why do I need people?" she demands.

This woman's features can seem carved in stone. As we sat above the Pacific watching the waves below, Denise and I discussed ALS, better known as Lou Gehrig's disease. The lady could laugh. Sometimes she would cry. We sat on a favorite wooden bench as she talked about where she might be taken next.

Far to the east, a graying middle-aged man explained that Jesus is going to cure him of a terminal illness and, yes, he is at peace. Buzz's smile lit the already bright outdoors as we crossed the town square at noon. He is a man of faith, a point of view that I strive to understand.

Buzz is struggling with non-Hodgkin's lymphoma, and deep into the fight of his life. Lymphoma used to be an automatic killer. The cancer cannot be cured but, for many, now can be managed.

"I would be angry," I tell him. "Why should I be angry?" he asked back. We had spent days hanging out in his little Indiana town, deep in the Bible Belt. His family and I had toured neighborhoods and gone to their church. I took Buzz at face value, and measured his quiet composure.

A thousand miles farther east and in separate cities,

two young people waited for another visit from me. Ben is a college student whose muscular dystrophy has left him in a wheelchair and in need of constant care. He struggles to make the present work as he stays sanguine about his uncertain future. The young man fights sickness and his fear of others.

Sarah almost died as an adolescent and was robbed of a colon by Crohn's disease. The siege continues. Confidence in her future ebbs as she bleeds from her gut. Her digestive tract continues to decay, and she fights to face her life. Ben and Sarah were toddlers when illness arrived. Each wears sickness from head to toe, and has never known health.

The diseases are different, the scars often similar. Both endure illnesses that grow only worse. One likely will leave before his time, the other, embrace a compromised life. "I am broken," Sarah says. "I will be alone," Ben predicts in a soft voice.

And there is the mountain man with the heart of a giant. A disease of the mind, bipolar disorder, had laid him low. Yet Larry has climbed high, his ascent greater than his fall. He is a better person for the journey. "We are all connected," he tells me, his beard white with the years.

These five have run the gauntlet, enduring a range of chronic illnesses. They are spectacular people whose willingness to share and give of themselves has been remarkable. The more I heard from each, the deeper grew my thoughts and connection with all of the others. And the better I understood myself.

I had spoken of each to the others, and their mutual fascination was not idle. We understood that we are all traveling the same highway and finally our ragtag army of the wounded had to meet, to talk and share.

What a wild thought, though we had to make it happen. We would connect the dots together in one place. They were so ready, longing to touch and be touched. Angels flew close. Wheels turned. They packed their belongings and their stories, crossed the country and converged.

The setting was the Harvard Club in downtown Boston. The space had seen better days, as had we all. This club was a caricature of itself, a monument to the privilege of another era. Entitlement was sewn into the upholstery. But this slowly gathering group was so un-Harvard; certainly there is no privilege in being sick.

If these were strangers, their presence was anything but strange. Every pore in that gilded room was open for business.

Ben sat tall in his wheelchair, shaking hands with Buzz. Black was meeting white, youth, middle-age. Ben is a college student, Buzz a working stiff. Muscular dystrophy is a disease of the young. Lymphoma had struck a man simply struggling for the chance to grow old.

Denise was among the last to show at the dinner, though she had been the first to venture into Boston the night before. California to New England had been a trek. Tonight, the little lady led with her walker, pushing forward as she said hello to Sarah. Smiles did not waver.

I had imagined this meeting for two years. Here, we would eat and drink, stand or sit, just hang out together to share. Something of great value would emerge. Of that I was certain.

My faltering eyes scanned the room. Only Larry was

missing in action. For a second I wondered if he was in trouble but then realized that I was guilty of believing the tired stereotype so many people have about bipolar disorder. In fact, Larry is grounded and steady, and has become my touchstone for evaluating everyone's behavior, including my own. Then Larry arrived.

Now it was time to go to work. The group had assembled. Some were surrounded by family. Others had brought only spouses, a parent, or a child. Only Denise had traveled alone. Our hosts were faculty members at Harvard Medical School. Their agenda was to give voice to patients and to encourage medical students to see their mission as treating whole people, not simply their diseases.

All of us carried stories about our experiences as patients in the world of medicine. Our mandate was to open a dialogue with future physicians about how to relate to the human being in the next bed.

For the sick, living among the healthy is no piece of cake. Empathy is in short supply. Daily brushes with public ignorance and indifference and the stigma of being sick in a society that worships health, brand and define us. Our group had so much to share.

First, we met privately. The following day we addressed the medical school community. No one in our group had played in this league before, yet all of us would prove willing and able to go to bat for our beliefs.

Clinical concerns had no place at our meeting. Those topics have their own home in worn volumes on shelves at medical schools everywhere. Too often, though, institutions of learning and doctors fail to widen the lens beyond the clinical. That may explain why doctors tend to see us as pages in those texts, notes in their charts. But that day at Harvard, we were people. We would offer living, breathing, rolling, walking, talking, stumbling stories of illness. Each of us has a take on surviving sickness, not to mention on the doctors who treat us. That material will not be found in those thick books on the shelves.

Chronic conditions become more common with age. According to the Centers for Disease Control, more than 80 percent of Americans over the age of sixty-five suffer from at least one chronic problem. Another 50 percent live with two.

America's health is deteriorating, a new fact of long life. We are fast becoming the oldest population in the history of the country, and the numbers of the stricken only grow. While the diseases differ, the emotional fallout from illness bears remarkable similarities.

For one moment, our small group would stand together. With separate stories, we would find unity. All of us had offered up intimate details of our struggles for this book. Now the youngest doctors could look deep into our eyes and hear the timbre of the voices to measure the pain.

Know this. Ninety million Americans battle chronic illnesses every day.

Welcome to your future.

two

Denise Glass

Fighting for Control

DENISE GLASS'S VOICE was slurred and strained, as if she had to deliberate each syllable before it could be uttered. By now, our long-distance conversations regularly left me thinking that mere talking must be exhausting for her. Her phone call on this autumn day was breathy and urgent, betraying her need to clear the air about some issue.

"Richard, I have to ask you something. I want you to tell me the truth," she instructed. "You keep saying not to pick you up at LAX," the airline code for Los Angeles International. "Are you afraid to ride with me because I have ALS?"

Silence. I thought I detected an implicit accusation in her question. "No, Denise," I replied slowly, feeling my way along. "I just did not want to inconvenience you." I stopped. "And besides, why would I worry about speed-

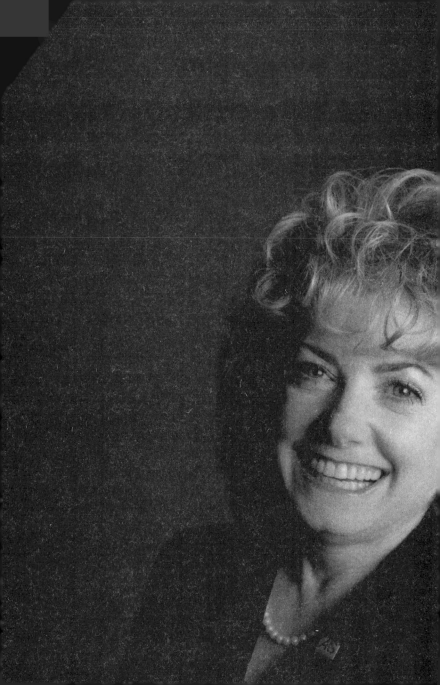

ing along the Ventura Freeway in a van, going eighty miles an hour, maybe, sitting in the front seat next to a tiny woman who can barely see over the wheel but is driving, and who, by the way, has ALS? I mean, what could go wrong?"

Another silence. This one had me worrying that I might have gone too far this time. Denise and I had been talking with increasing frequency and intensity on the phone. And our long-distance dance was drawing us ever closer to a painful reality. We had to meet face-to-face. Only then might the walls come tumbling down.

Maybe this woman did not find my remark so funny. Laughter does not come easily in a conversation about ALS. I well understood why Denise would be defensive, would be checking her radar for indications of condescension or just plain ignorance.

A familiar easy giggle across thousands of miles carried the reassuring answer: I had not destroyed our evolving relationship with my clumsy attempt at using humor to defuse the awkward moment, something I had been doing for so many years in dealing with my own struggles with illness in an indifferent world.

But would Denise rise to the occasion? "Yeah," she got out laboriously. "Who knows what will happen with me behind the wheel?"

In the back of my mind, I wondered the same. ALS was new to me, with one more letter of the alphabet and, in most cases, many times the pain of MS. Denise behind the wheel did seem slightly scary. "Well," I remarked, "I figure you know what you are doing, and I assume you have no plans to kill yourself."

Again there was a pause before her flat reply: "Yet."

To that, I said nothing. Yet.

I ARRIVED AT LAX in warm autumn sunshine a few weeks later. The temperate clime was a welcome contrast to the parade of dank, cloudy days at home in New York. "Don't bother coming inside the terminal," I had told Denise. "I'll meet you outside baggage claim. It's a hassle inside, and you'll never get past security without a ticket."

"Yes, I will," she answered sharply. "Just leave it to me."

Fine. I was learning not to argue with her, at least about airplanes and cars. "I, of course, will not know you," I pointed out.

"What should we do?" Denise asked.

"Just stand at the gate, holding a large balloon," I suggested with a self-conscious laugh.

When I emerged through the gate into a moving mass of humanity, walking shakily on legs that too often seem part-time partners, I heard a soft voice saying something slowly and none too crisply. "Richard," I heard again. I looked to my left and came face-to-face with a large blue balloon. I cast my eyes down a ways. There was a pretty blonde with a large, pretty smile.

"Denise" was all I could muster in my halting, hoarse voice. We each seemed suddenly shy, despite our frequent telephone conversations. Here was my mail-order bride in the flesh, there to greet me after my long push west. Two thoughts flashed across my mind: Denise Glass seems tough and fragile at the same time. And, boy, is she short.

Denise, then forty-seven, stands at just four feet, eleven inches, but she can carry herself as if the world were hers.

I eyed her tentatively as we began our trek out. She pushed her way slowly but determinedly through the crowds, down the concourse, and through baggage claim, to the parking lot.

Her gait was as deliberate as her speech. The little lady's energy was high, as were her spirits. I silently smiled at the sight we must have made: a tiny woman hobbling uncertainly on a pink flowered cane, keeping apace of a half-blind giant shuffling along with his plain wooden cane.

As we moved along, Denise laid out a schedule for my visit. First, we were going to pick up some lunch. Then we were going to talk. "Denise, I plan to invade your privacy," I had warned her in one of our phone conversations. "I plan to ask you a lot of prying and personal questions about your life. I want to hear your story."

There was the usual pause. I could sense her mouth gearing up to manufacture words. "Come out to California," she had replied with a soft chuckle, though even getting out the name of her state seemed tough. "You don't scare me. I am ready for you."

Denise was living in Calabasas. This community of more than twenty-five thousand sits in the craggy Santa Monica Mountains northwest of Los Angeles. The area has grown wildly as a suburb of L.A., with traffic streaming up and down near the California coastline.

Still, there are the parks and hiking trails coexisting with shopping malls and apartment complexes. Calabasas was an ideal base for a Californian like Denise, who thrived on the outdoors. Since the onset of her illness, nature had also become a refuge from her radically changing health.

We drove to a favorite spot high above the Pacific and

climbed up a short trail. Sitting on a wooden bench above the crashing waves, we began to talk. When we wandered too far into the future, the conversation came too close for comfort. Denise switched gears and tried to talk about me. Questions about the final stages of ALS were asked, and Denise became vague, occasionally just turning silent, as if unplugged.

Gradually, I was getting glimpses of a very different Denise from the woman on the phone. Hiding is easier when the other person cannot see, and now I was in her face. The calm, in-control woman she put on display for me and most of the world was not so much at peace. Composure had taken up residence on the surface. Just below, a cauldron was bubbling.

"It is all gone," she said in a broken whisper, letting the tears trickle as she described how ALS had robbed her of her dreams and transformed her life. And she spoke of an empathy that had been born. "I see life differently now. When I see someone in a wheelchair or on a walker, I want to go up and hug them and say, 'I am sorry you are sick. I know how you feel.'"

Denise has become a raw, frayed nerve. "I feel for them and for me. I know I am going to be there. I am frightened. I try not to think about it. But it is becoming more and more of a reality now. The disease moved slowly for a while, but now it is progressing. I am falling more now. It is frightening," she repeated with a faint quiver. I envy her emotion. Mine is buried who knows where.

Denise's cell phone rang suddenly. Would we drive to Beverly Hills to visit another ALS patient and his family? a mother wondered. Denise turned to me. I shrugged. "We will do whatever you want," I said. "This guy is in lock-down," she told me in a soft voice. I nodded blankly, not knowing what that meant. The timbre of her voice gave me pause.

We headed south along the Pacific. ALS seemed an ugly subject for such a beautiful setting. We drove into Beverly Hills, turning corners past manicured lawns and large homes that marked lives of privilege. Except for the place whose driveway we turned up.

We parked the car and walked into a spacious ranch house, where we were greeted by an older couple. Almost immediately, we were led into an adjoining room and I saw what Denise so feared. Now would come my first contact with the terrifying cruelty, if not certainty, of this neurode-generative disease.

Neil just lay there. He was a man in his forties, alone in a hospital bed placed in a well-appointed living room. He looked healthy, pink-skinned and bright-eyed. But he was inanimate, a statue in repose. Neil's limbs were immobile, his lips still, without a twitch or quiver. His eyes were un-blinking. Every five minutes, a soft alarm sounded, a signal for a full-time nurse to put drops into his frozen eyes. A feeding tube kept nourishment coming, a ventilator sent oxygen pumping to make breathing possible.

Neil had been an academic ophthalmologist, a well-educated man with a vigorous body and an agile brain. His fertile mind remained intact, but now was imprisoned in a motionless body. Total lockdown had lasted four years. Neil had had only limited speech and use of his limbs for almost four years before that.

The young physician's only means of communication

through the lockdown years had been by polygraph, a lie-detector machine, whose electrodes were hooked up to his body. A companion or visitor would say something to Neil or point to a number or a letter of the alphabet to slowly spell out a word, then wait for Neil's involuntary response to be translated by the machine.

This had become a private language that only Neil's close family could understand. His needs and wants were laboriously, though reliably, determined by this long process. Both parents said they had developed their own instincts, a sixth sense for what Neil needed. Neil could communicate that something was wrong. His mother said he diagnosed his own complications and always was right. "Neil still is a great doctor," she told me.

Neil resided with his parents, who were retired and ready to take on his care. Neil's wife and two teenage sons lived in the neighborhood and made frequent visits. "Neil is watching those beautiful children grow up," his father said with satisfaction.

A man cut down in his prime, a part-time family, and communication by committee seemed unacceptable to me. In the end, interacting through lie-detector tests is a guessing game as much as a science and certainly a scene right out of the movies. Why was this poor guy's life being strung along? I could not imagine myself wanting to continue on in that situation. Is that presumptuous? I wondered.

"We communicate with Neil and know he wants to go on," his father, a retired surgeon, assured me. "Neil's brothers wonder about keeping him alive, but he is clear. He wants to live." Neil had been hospitalized with renal failure, his kidneys shutting down. "Neil made the decision himself to go on dialysis."

Neil's ability to reach out to others had been evolving. The family was working with two corporations deep in the space-age communications business. Their specialists were using the ailing doctor as a guinea pig. Infrared light was beamed to his forehead, measuring blood flow in the brain. "Neil can tell us a lot about his life."

"They are perfecting programs to control devices. There are robotic arms. This has worked in the lab," Neil's mother said.

"Does this give you hope?"

"Oh, yes. This may be around the corner." Neil's mother looked away. "Neil knows this may not happen in his lifetime, but we have to help others."

As I took in the spectacle, Denise was taking slow steps back, seeking distance, it seemed, as a defense mechanism. She stayed away from Neil's line of sight, longing to be invisible. For her, Neil's bed was a world away. Her thoughts remained her silent possession.

I took a breath and walked to the edge of the bed to begin a one-way conversation with this man. I told him about the book and my life, my hopes for reaching out to patients of all diseases. The ventilator offered the only sound in the room as I paused. Neil's gaze was steady. I looked into his eyes and imagined he understood. Denise continued to say nothing.

My eyes were opened on this afternoon. I saw ALS more clearly in one hour than most witness in a lifetime. Probabilities, perhaps inevitabilities, were screaming into my head. This was the real thing. Southern California sure looked different from this block of Beverly Hills. "This is a freaking wax museum," echoed through my head.

As we pulled away from Neil's home, I looked over at Denise. She sat silent behind the wheel, eyes fixed forward, just staring. I could not look at her again until we had traveled a good distance. When Neil died almost three years later, Denise says she gasped before the inevitability of it all set in. She knew she was on the same road.

EARLY THE NEXT morning after meeting Neil, Denise picked me up from my motel and we drove to one more park. We walked to a bench in a quiet corner, took out supplies and prepared to talk. As I fiddled with a tape recorder, I looked up and saw Denise laying out a line of carefully sliced lemon wedges. She seemed to labor casually, forming a neat row but making no mention of the task.

What an odd ritual, I thought, lemons at the ready. We began another difficult conversation. Emotions skyrocket when talk turns to threatening illness. As our conversation grew intense, Denise became teary-eyed and soon began to cry. Without a word, she picked up a lemon wedge and sucked on it, continuing where she had paused.

"Denise," I interrupted, "what are you doing?"

"When I cry, the mucus builds up and can block my breathing," she explained in a thick, halting voice between sobs.

"Is that clogging dangerous?"

"Oh, yeah," she sort of said. "The lemon cuts the mucus. It unclogs my throat."

From that moment, lemon wedges were on the menu for our meetings. And whenever Denise began to choke on her mucus, we repeated a mantra. "Go suck a lemon," we would say in unison.

The ritual of the lemons revealed Denise's strong streak of self-reliance. When a meeting was planned and the day was young, she could be found at her kitchen counter, preparing her survival kit. She would talk to herself, quietly rattling off what would be needed that day. Preparing the lemons was her calm before the storm.

The lemons also gave evidence of how careful Denise had had to become. She lived on a tightrope. She ate and drank selectively as a matter of routine, avoiding a growing list of foods and beverages that might choke and kill her.

Personal destruction, indeed disintegration, is what ALS—amyotrophic lateral sclerosis—is all about. This neurodegenerative disease is commonly called Lou Gehrig's disease because that's easier to say and sounds less foreboding. Lou Gehrig, the 1930s Yankee baseball star, was an American icon, and putting his name on the disease that killed him placed the illness front and center in public view.

But ALS is not sport. The illness is as bad as it gets, bringing on terror, not simply fear. The disease usually strikes people between the ages of forty and seventy. As many as thirty-thousand Americans, more men than women, are afflicted at any given time. Every ninety minutes, someone is diagnosed with or dies from ALS. There seems to be an increased rate of ALS among veterans of the 1991 Gulf War.

At first, I felt a shortness of breath just being in Denise's company. Sheer anxiety, I decided. What do you say to someone who is going to disintegrate and die? A lot, as it turned out. And Denise had a lot to say back.

With ALS, there can be no realistic optimism. There is only the hope to live a little longer and be spared the worst horror before the inevitable slide down. What is that like? How does anyone handle such a grim future? ALS offers no more than a journey with a most certain end and no knowable schedule. That is true of life, but ALS accelerates the scheduled departure considerably.

When Denise and I met, she had been living with the disease for five years. Her ALS is known as nonhereditary sporadic ALS, a form that randomly strikes any person and any part of the body. Denise's ALS first attacked the bulbar region of the brain, damaging her speech and her ability to swallow, but eventually, in a process called limbonset, it journeyed down her spine to affect her arms and her legs and points between. There is no cure for this, no treatment. Nothing.

People with ALS survive, on average, four to five years after diagnosis. Some live a shorter time, others significantly longer. "Stephen Hawking, the scientist, has had ALS for thirty years," Denise pointed out, reassuring me and herself. "A woman in our ALS chapter has had it for twenty. Mine is slow. It could speed up. Who knows?"

HOWEVER LONG HER life, this, certainly, was not the life Denise was raised to expect. She grew up in Woodland Hills, a middle-class suburb of Los Angeles. "We had a very normal family," she said. "I have parents and a sister and two brothers. I am the second child, which is different than the first."

How? I asked, a middle child myself and instinctively knowing the answer.

"My sister got the new stuff. I got hand-me-downs. My mom sews, and she made me clothes, which was good because I was so small." In other ways, too, Denise felt she did not keep pace with her siblings. The family was big on achievement and success. "I always felt I was less of a student," she remembered. "School was hard for me."

Still, she harbored traditional ambitions and hopes. "That you go to college and work, and you meet a nice guy, and get married, and have kids, you know, the fantasy. And I did try to live it. I went to college and could not wait to start working." She looked around her cluttered kitchen. We were back at the house after a frenetic day of running around L.A. "I moved out and was on my own at twenty-one and worked my brains off. I would always give one hundred and ten percent."

The fantasy faded for Denise, as happens with everyone. Time and experience interceded. She did not make it to a full college degree. Her career did not measure up to what she wanted. She had to handle a failed marriage and, more devastating, a pregnancy that ended in miscarriage and a hysterectomy. The dream had paled but was not snuffed out, until ALS came her way.

Denise had bounced around, changing jobs with some frequency. She was a legal secretary here, an executive assistant somewhere else. She also had human resources credentials on her résumé. Then Denise decided it was time for a change. She created her own business, building a list of clients for whom she provided all three services. Ultimately, she did not take to the grind and retreated back to the cocoon of corporate life as an executive assistant.

Late in 2000, Denise began to notice that her speech had slowed and swallowing was becoming difficult. "I did not do anything for a while," she said. "I told no one, but the difference was becoming obvious. My family asked, 'What is wrong with you? Why is your speech so slow?' I said, 'I don't know. Everything feels the same, but it is slow.'"

Denise's internist referred her to a neurologist, who examined her but showed little concern. The doctor ordered an MRI, later announcing his diagnosis. "'Stress,' he told me. 'You need to get the stress out of your life. Get rid of it.' He was the doctor. Who was I to question the diagnosis?" Denise may have been in the early stages of denial, a definite possibility since she might have known better, given a personal experience.

Only three years earlier, she had watched her boss, Harry, succumb in slow-motion to ALS. "His speech was not as slow as mine," Denise remembered, "but it was more garbled." As months passed, Harry's symptoms grew worse. No one, least of all Harry, seemed to know what was wrong.

"Harry thought, 'Oh, maybe something is the matter with my jaw,'" Denise recalled. Based on her account of events, Harry seemed reluctant to learn more. "He was a lawyer and had to go to court, and he sounded like he was drunk." That should wake a guy up. "Well, Harry finally ended up going to the Mayo Clinic, and then he got the diagnosis."

Denise seemed to be following Harry's lead, looking

away and denying the possibilities. "When I started notic-ing my speech and my swallowing and having problems with my saliva, Harry did come to mind right away." And? "And I would think, 'Nah, it cannot be ALS. It can't.'"

"So were you in denial?" I asked.

"It was wishful thinking, I guess," she replied.

"Not denial?"

Denise paused. "Not denial."

Right.

Doctors kept offering Denise hideouts. A year after seeing the neurologist, and with her difficulties only in-creasing, her family began to wonder if the problems were all in her head. Denise again called her internist. He re-ferred her to another neurologist.

The second specialist did another MRI and a swallow study. Myasthenia gravis, he informed her. "He said he was sure, and he gave me medication." And then? "The medication made me so sick that I had a very hard time swallowing it," she said.

Denise was now zero for two. She was being taunted by a cruel disease and had the Keystone Docs on her case.

"How do you account for these misdiagnoses?"

"They were wrong," she shot back, "dead wrong."

"Were you angry?"

"This is not uncommon for ALS," she observed.

"Yeah," I said. "Were you angry?"

"Yes."

"It is very hard to diagnose ALS," Denise said. "It is not a common ailment."

"When did you figure it out?" I asked.

"When the medicine for the myasthenia gravis did not

work, I thought of Harry again. And I just knew I had ALS. And it was getting worse."

When she confronted her internist for the third time and told him her belief, he sent her to an ALS specialist at UCLA. "She is a wonderful woman with a heart of gold," Denise said. "She had me do a swallow study, but on video, not one where they take still pictures and cannot see anything going down."

Denise got the official confirmation of ALS in August 2001. "I went to UCLA with my parents."

"It is a death sentence to tell you that you have ALS," the doctor told her. "I cannot tell you any more about how long you have. We cannot do anything for you. Just try and stay as healthy as you can," the doc advised. "Eat as much as you can," she went on. "Do not lose weight."

Denise was being advised to gaze into the future and prepare herself. "When the ALS progresses, a feeding tube is necessary, and you automatically lose weight." Denise was choked with emotion as she finished her account of the diagnosis. She had to pause. "Go suck a lemon," I suggested, not knowing what else to say. And she did just that.

I looked back to the moment of my diagnosis with MS, a life sentence at hard labor compared to Denise's death sentence with no appeal. It was clear that this woman could not get beyond the mere fact of the diagnosis. At the instant of hearing a neurologist's words and knowing my own fate, hours were crammed into the blink of an eye. I saw the rest of my life and played out my fears. I made a decision about how I was going to react. Did Denise have a similar response? I wondered. "Not really," she answered with no embellishment.

For her, shock shut out thought. Even though the doctor's information was what Denise was expecting, the words hit with force. "It was like the doctor punched a fist into my gut and all the air came out of my diaphragm." Denise looked down. "I was, like, gasping for air."

"And your gut reaction?"

"I was pissed off and angry. When I came out of the building, there were these big plates of glass, and all I wanted to do was punch my fist right through them. I could not get past that anger for a while." For some of us, it never passes. Working through the white heat, traveling past the moment of rage, takes an acquired skill.

That night, after the awful news was delivered, Denise sat with her roommate, Peggy, who also had worked for Harry. Denise fixed on the final piece of advice the doctor had given her. "Listen. This part is very important," Denise said, repeating what she had been told. "'Get rid of stress,' she had told me. Go and have fun. Enjoy your life. Travel while you can. Be active. Do not sit and dwell on this, or you will go into a depression, which will have a snowball effect and make everything you face only worse.'"

In a state of high emotion, the two women drew up a list of activities and goals Denise was drawn to, adventures beyond her everyday life. They named continents and countries Denise wanted to visit, sights to be seen before her body betrayed her. "It was difficult." Denise recalled. Difficult and very emotional.

"We were tearful, actually," Denise slowly recounted. "I had to admit that my life was very boring. All I did was work, work, work, or be with my two kitty-cats, who were the loves of my life. Stained Glass and Crystal Glass were their names."

Denise got creative. "I always wanted to go a hundred twenty miles per hour in a Mercedes," she said, chuckling softly.

"Did you do it?"

"Yeah, I did."

"How did you pull that off?"

"I cannot tell you when or with whom it happened. I am sworn to secrecy. And it was not a Mercedes sports car, it was a Porsche." For Denise, the prospect of dying was beginning to clarify how she wanted to live. "It made me get off my duff," she observed. Her life shifted away from caution.

"I decided to do the hardest things first," she said, "because I saw my body changing." Denise packed a bag and traveled to Anchorage for the Fur Rondy winter carnival. She journeyed north again to photograph the California and Oregon coastlines. She enrolled in clown school. Then came the kicker: Antarctica.

"I am going on a cruise to Antarctica," she announced early in our relationship, her excitement palpable. "I have to see the penguins and seals on those icebergs before I die."

"Are you serious?" I shot back, sounding disapproving, even to myself. My tongue had been quicker than my brain, my knee-jerk judgment as bad as everyone else's. My instant challenge betrayed the stupid assumption of recklessness I so resent coming my way from others.

I was selling Denise short because she was sick. What a jerk I am, was all I could think. I am the guy who covered a few wars for television news when I could see only a few vague shapes across a street. And I was preaching the virtues of conservative common sense. "Relax," Denise had said softly. "It will be great falling off an iceberg."

My footing recovered, I tried again. "Why exactly are you doing this, Denise?" I asked more reasonably. "This seems as if it will be a very arduous trip." Denise inhaled deeply. "I have to see those penguins and seals with my own eyes. I want to stand on an ice floe and watch the sunset." I do not expect to die of MS. For Denise, sunset must take on new meaning. "Richard, I need to do this."

In an article for the *ALS Society Journal,* Denise identified the emotional fuel that propelled her to the end of the earth. "As my ALS progresses, my left hand and leg are becoming weaker. That has made me more determined than ever. I have to pursue my dreams."

She sold her condo—the stairs were increasingly hard to maneuver, and it was the right time for a change—and used the proceeds to finance her journey. I rode around L.A. with Denise a month before she was to head south while she picked up warm clothes and boots for the weeks she would be spending above deck and below zero.

Anticipation ran high. "It is the whole thought of being down there and doing the trip with my ALS," she exclaimed in a breathy voice. "If I did not have ALS, I would not be going there. There would have been no time or incentive to live the way you are supposed to," she explained at a busy intersection. "I would be too busy living a life I did not care about. I have changed. I'm doing things I would never have done."

The trip was rough. Denise flew to Miami and caught another plane to Ushuaia, Argentina. She traveled by car to the shores of the Drake Passage, where the Pacific and Atlantic oceans merge. The ship, *Explorer 2*, was waiting. Safe in her cabin, Denise wept with relief and excitement. Once under sail, the seas were harrowing. At one point, twenty-five-foot swells and seventy-mile-an-hour winds kept Denise in her bed for almost a day.

The continent at the bottom of the earth became a metaphor for Denise's struggle. The landscape is overwhelming, wide, and bleak. The trek across is lonely and dangerous. Antarctica accounts for 10 percent of the earth's surface and contains 90 percent of its ice. This would prove a hostile venue for proving a point.

But the strain of the long journey was worth it. "Seeing the tabular icebergs, magnificent Antarctica sunsets, were breathtaking," she e-mailed. At four o'clock one morning, they boarded Zodiac boats to go ashore. "I was walking on the beach with penguins by my side. I was crying because it was overwhelming and I still could not believe I was there." The mere fact of the trip meant as much to her as the splendor.

Denise understood that she could not conquer ALS, so she traded that impossible challenge for a rigorous task she could complete. As a sojourner below the equator, she survived a strenuous challenge and could claim victory over that. The experience was part exploration, part mind game.

"It took a disease to open my eyes and force me to muster the courage to do something." Denise chuckled softly. "I did not know I had it in me."

"Any regrets?"

"No way," Denise snapped. "Not a day goes by when I do not think of Antarctica and what I did."

"And you learned from the trip?"

"Yeah. Every day, live your life and live your dreams."

IF THIS WERE a movie, we would shoot a slow fade on Denise, standing taller than she can, triumphant and happy on the ice floes. She would appear in the shadow of the craggy, wild mountains of Antarctica. Real life tells a more prosaic story. It is a much smaller life filled with fears and daily frustrations.

ALS makes swallowing difficult, and Denise has had to overhaul her eating habits. "I have to think through every meal," she said in a weary voice. It had become a time-consuming routine, a "pain in the ass," according to her. Dairy and spicy sauces are banned; they could gag and choke her. Steak, vegetables, and fruits have to be cut up in small pieces to avoid the same. Dry and crumbly bread and cheeses are cut out altogether. Denise drinks water at room temperature with no ice. Cold constricts the throat. The H_2O is sipped through a straw.

"Can you eat anything halfway edible and interesting?"

"I had French toast just this morning," she told me with no hint of humor. Apparently, food is no laughing matter. "I drenched it in syrup so I could just swallow it."

"Any other recipes?"

"Hamburgers are always good." Pause. "But it is always with a lot of ketchup and a glass of water right there. Look," she said suddenly. "I do what is needed to get the stuff down."

What Denise chooses to eat is but the beginning. "The way I sleep in bed. If I am lying flat, I choke. It is hard to get in and out of bed. It is getting harder." It takes constant focus just to get through another day. "The way I get dressed in the morning is a contest with myself," she said, describing her contortions. "Standing on one leg to put on a sock, those days are over. Even putting on underwear, I have to sit down. You have to think of a way to get your foot in."

The exasperation in her voice as she described the daily grind was clear. "Everything we all take for granted has been taken away. Now I live a different life." Every minute of this woman's day is centered on ALS. It is the only game in town. "Oh, yes," came quick corroboration. "Walking down the street and not falling is big. I get tired of constantly keeping ALS in the front of my mind. But you've got to. All I think about is figuring out ways to keep surviving, just continuing to live."

Just the thought of this makes me crave a stiff drink. "Oh, and I miss my pinot grigio like you cannot believe," Denise groaned, laughing and choking slightly at the same time. Wine makes her gag, but for a treat on a New Year's Eve she allowed herself a small glass diluted so much that it tasted like grape-flavored water. "It's almost not worth it," she said glumly.

Denise brings a level of discipline to her struggle that has evaded me in mine. I miss by a mile. MS, too, makes swallowing difficult, but I have no patience for sensible, healthful calculations. My internist once told me he figured that sooner or later I would choke to death because I was not smart enough to chew my food thoroughly or slow down.

Denise knows and does precisely what is good for her. I tend to do the opposite, defying common sense, jaywalking with seriously impaired vision across busy New York intersections.

Immaturity beckoning? Perhaps. I think of those acts as choices, a stubborn refusal to make even small concessions to a disease I do not respect. Denise has to respect ALS; the illness is just too dangerous to defy. Defiance may be a luxury belonging to those who believe they will survive.

As her body weakened, Denise resorted first to using a cane, then a walker. The stick had a festive air with its pastel flowers, but the walker was a grim emblem of disintegration. Denise had to give up the two-story rented house she moved into after she sold her condo because she could no longer navigate the stairs. She moved to a modest ranch house on a quiet street just off the Ventura freeway. Her van sits high enough from the pavement so that getting in and out is a struggle. Her own wheels, parked outside that house, are her last hope for independence.

People park under Denise's skin with relative ease. Assumption and attitude make her crazy, and she gets plenty of both. "I get very frustrated with the world," she announced one day. "People will not take the time to understand and be compassionate. As soon as I open my mouth at a store or anywhere, people turn around and look at me like, 'Are you mentally retarded?' 'Are you deaf and trying to speak?'"

Denise is most self-conscious about the slurred speech that is characteristic of bulbar ALS. She has learned what my less-pronounced slur from MS taught me long ago: people jump to conclusions. "Are you drunk?" becomes the common query. "Of course, I do not drink," Denise complained. "People do not know that, and they assume the worst." She paused. "You know, it is so hard not to flip people off." Welcome to a world of ignorance. "People also assume I had a stroke, especially because of the cane." She laughed ruefully. "I wish it was just a stroke."

Denise was getting worked up, pausing only for the laborious process of breathing. "When you're out, people tend to gravitate to the one who is not ill and ignore the sick person. This is how people respond to me, even though I always will be mentally intact."

"How does that make you feel?" I asked.

"I guess I am used to it." Or not.

"I think people are stupid and condescending," I said. "What can they be thinking?"

"That you are not normal, so get out of here." Denise believed judgment was instant and harsh. "You are not normal, so I do not need to communicate with you. You are not worthy of my time."

"People say that?"

"No. I see their faces. And they turn away."

Denise has found perspective over the years. "I think, Do I want them to remember me because I flip them off? No. So what I say loudly is this: 'My speech is slow. I have Lou Gehrig's disease, ALS. My mind is fine. I am not mentally retarded. In fact, I am probably smarter than you.'"

Denise worked up a head of steam. "When they have been really rude, I say, 'Please be patient. I know what I'm going to say. I just cannot speak it. So let me know if you do not understand.' I say this all the time."

"That's polite."

"I can be polite." Pause. "Sometimes."

The communication gap is daunting. It reared its head when Denise came to visit in New York. Canceled planes, hours of delays, and a long flight eventually dumped an exhausted Denise at JFK airport late one stormy night. The terminal was nearly empty and when she arranged for her car service, the cranky airline employees certainly did not make her feel welcome to New York.

Her surly driver got lost. Denise's tiredness had long passed her anger. Always one step ahead, she pulled out handwritten notes she had prepared during the flight and gave them to the driver. The small pieces of paper named the Times Square hotel where she was staying and described just what her problem was.

"Can't speak," the note read. "I have ALS, Lou Gehrig's disease." The driver did not want to deal with her. "He just looked away."

"Weren't you angry?"

She sighed loudly. "Yeah, but what is the point?"

I said nothing.

Denise cannot accept that people can act horribly. She expects better and cannot shrug off the disappointment. She takes ugly encounters personally, as if insult and injury are fired only at her.

"One night, I called a very large electronics store to find out the cost of something and their return policy. I called six times and kept getting the runaround on their recording machine." She was getting upset just telling this story. "Finally I got Edmund." Her lip quivered as she continued. "Edmund went to ask someone, and he left the phone open, meaning he did not put it on hold. He said to the other salesperson, 'I have this old lady who is drunk on the phone. She is screaming at me and trying to find out our return policy.' Then I said, 'Okay, Edmund. Next time you want to bad-mouth a customer, you need to put the phone on hold. And furthermore, I have a fatal disease, and it is called ALS, Lou Gehrig's disease. It has affected my speech. But believe me, my brain is better than yours.'"

Denise relishes the small victory. "When I have to deal with the public, my anger comes out because they are ignorant. They do not know what I'm going through."

I hate to say this, Denise, but welcome to the real world. No one wants to know.

People with busy lives do not have time to know and do not want to care. Folks out there do not feel comfortable getting involved with people who are sick. They will write checks to charities and put money in the basket at church. That is impersonal giving, sympathy from a distance. It keeps consciences as well as hands clean and sickness far away.

Those who suffer sickness learn to put on a brave front. Sometimes this has less to do with the steel of a strong spine than the desire to avoid dealing with the subject at all. Why bother? People do not want to know, anyway.

The most insincere question in the language has become, "How are you?" In my own life, I have become inured to it. People really do not want to know and inquire under the assumption that no one will be rude enough to actually answer the question honestly. I ignore the façade of concern.

Screw the positive attitude, anyway. Give me anger and frustration anytime. Those are honest emotions. We are taught that they are unhealthy barriers to acceptance and peace. I do not think so, because acceptance is poison and peace comes only in a permanent, horizontal position. I wanted to talk about anger, and Denise did not need to be pressed.

"Yeah, and I am pissed off as hell that I have ALS and have to deal with it," Denise allowed. "And then I think, what is getting angry going to do for me? Nothing."

"Isn't there something to be said for releasing steam?"

"Yeah, but what can I do about having ALS? Nothing. Then why be angry? You'd better accept it."

"You cannot be serious. Does that work?" I asked.

"No," Denise half-laughed, suggesting that nothing about this was funny.

There is no silver bullet. "When this happened," she said. "I was given a phrase: DABDA." The acronym for Dr. Elisabeth Kübler-Ross's seminal emotional stages of dying: Denial. Anger. Bargaining. Depression. Acceptance.

"I do not mean to quarrel with Dr. Kübler-Ross," I said, "but I do not buy her roadmap for coping. Her order of emotions is off, and I doubt that each flows automatically into the next."

I have dabbled in denial on my journey and have hit the brakes after anger. I can slow or even stop that anger after skidding, but I see nobody to bargain with. I have no time for depression, have avoided acceptance, which is tantamount to surrender. This leaves me to travel my own path, and I can live with that.

Did Denise find DABDA any more helpful than I had? "No," she answered quickly. Then her words softened. "In the beginning I was mad at everyone and everything. Then it evolved into being angry that I had to be the one to get ALS." She had ratcheted up just being mad. "Then I was back to 'Okay, I've had it.'"

"In other words, you were all over the map."

"Right."

Jerry Goldman, a Toronto newsman writing about his own reactions to having ALS, argued that Kübler-Ross missed a stage. "Actually, it's the first one you confront," he wrote on his website. "Shock. Bang! You have a disease and you're going to die. What! No, can't be. How did this happen? There must be a mistake. Holy crap, I'm gonna die? This is insane. I can't die. I don't want to die. And so on. I'M GONNA DIE."

"Oh yeah," Denise squealed over the phone when I read her Goldman's Internet outburst. "For me it was like that." She did not burn through the shock. "It comes back as a repeating bad dream. You do not forget the feeling. I still don't. Some days, on my down days, the shock does not go away."

"Will it ever?"

"I doubt it."

I asked her if she thought she would *ever* make peace with her fate.

"Probably not. I got cheated," she answered.

Does she even *want* to find peace?

"Why? What is the point?" she demanded. "Should I have it and be happy? Yeah, right."

I rest my case. Making peace with serious or hopeless illness should be reserved for priests and patients on bad TV shows. Acceptance is not a real-world concept. For me, a semi-vacant look is the best response to queries about making peace with illness. To make peace with an illness becomes appeasement. I need frustration and anger to keep me going. The bitter flailing at what I can no longer do with my body becomes an emotionally safer target than the illness itself.

I called Denise to ask if she understood what I meant by anger being converted to fuel for living and was taken aback by how subdued she seemed. "I fell last night," she told me. "I hurt my left side, my hip and butt," adding, "I am losing my balance. I have to go slower and think about what I am doing."

"Does that piss you off?" I asked.

"Yeah." She sighed. "What can I do? This is not me. It isn't. If you knew me before I was sick—this is not me."

"How does it make you feel?"

"It makes me angry." She paused. "I will never be normal again."

"And where does the anger fit in?" I prodded.

"Anger keeps me going and helps me and pushes me to prove to myself that I can still do everything I could, even though I cannot." I could hear her begin to weep softly. "I did not cry too much until I started talking to you."

Great.

I worry that this book is a cruel exercise because the mirror is held so close.

"I will never be able to run up and down the stairs again. Ever."

You and me both.

"Do you miss running?" she asked.

"I do," I told her. "A lot."

"You've had MS for so long." Denise was breathy. "This is new to me. You are used to it."

"Not really," I answered. And no, I said in my head, you never get used to it.

Running down the stairs is just a memory, I told Denise, realizing that the day before, I had stared at people going up and down stairs and wondered how they kept their balance without leaning on a rail or using a cane.

"When I fell, I did it on my cane," Denise offered. "It hurt."

"I find that what hurts is not being able even to imagine negotiating stairs without the cane."

Here is a little-known true fact. Sickness hurts, and not just emotionally. Everyday injuries, the contusions and cuts, sprains and scrapes, become the regular price for surviving another day. Legs are weak, balance gone. Mishaps are steady. Bruising the body injures the spirit. Get pissed at the symptoms and, in your head, keep a safe distance from the disease.

Anger becomes utilitarian. Letting off steam before there is an explosion allows us to continue the struggle, to focus emotional energy on how difficult our lives have become, not when they will end. The very fact of a disease that kills may be impossible to absorb, but bathing in mortality is no way to cleanse a troubled mind.

DENISE AND I were driving along a narrow road, winding our way through an arid canyon connecting Malibu with the hectic, wildly growing towns east of the mountains. I silently noted that Denise drove decisively, in firm control of her white van, even as her control over the rest of her life was ebbing.

"I do not want to talk about my family," she announced for the umpteenth time.

"Whatever," I said, as if this were the first time I had heard the remark.

"I just don't," she followed crisply, trying to slam a closed door. "It would upset them."

"They upset you," I responded. Denise lost interest in the conversation.

I did not get it. Every family has its baggage, but flesh and blood are everything. The DNA is there. Parents and siblings should offer solace and support. Since family seemed an explosive issue with Denise, I began with religion, the safer subject. "I am not an atheist," she said, "but religion is not a big part of my life." She shrugged as she drove. "I just do not feel it. I can be spiritually moved but not because of any religion."

Organized religion and spirituality can have little to do with each other. "When I say, 'Oh, my God,' who knows what god I am talking about?" She said, laughing. Denise is a Jew, though hardly observant. Occasionally, she attends a nondenominational church with a spiritual emphasis. I think in some circles that is known as Religion Lite.

God may be missing in action on Denise's personal battleground, and so, it seems, are her parents and siblings. There had been no sense in our conversations on coping of her family having a meaningful role in her drama. I had heard nothing to suggest that her family even stands on the stage. "I do not want you to write about that," she told me repeatedly. Fine, I would say back—that is, until finally I realized her family *did* play an important role.

Denise's disappointment, even anger, toward her family was neither veiled nor vague. The familial response to her illness, she said outright, was consistently cold and disengaged. They did not seem to care to know about her disease or understand her ordeal. Denise's observations about family came at awkward times, when we were arriving somewhere, with little opportunity for follow-up. Who had pushed whom away was not clear.

Geographic distance seemed hardly the issue. Her parents, Selma and Al, live in a retirement village in the California desert near Palm Springs, a few hours by car from Denise. Her older sister, Lori, lives with her family near Denise. She also has two brothers, who live in other states, and whom she rarely mentioned. Other families manage greater distances, and always there is the option of moving closer to one another. So why did Denise's family seem to be missing? "I just want to meet your family," I kept saying.

Denise had been given permission to take me to an ALS Association training session for spouses and partners of newly diagnosed ALS patients. These meetings usually are private because participants are so vulnerable and their emotions so openly displayed. We sat in the back and tried to blend in.

The session was raw and riveting. The newly inducted caregivers seemed predictably bewildered, deer in the headlights. The caseworker leading the seminar was advising these individuals of the physical horrors they could expect to encounter in their loved ones. This compassionate woman laid out the psychological needs that probably would present themselves in the not-so-distant future.

The scene was sobering. I watched Denise watch the new class of suffering spouses. I wondered what was going through her head as she contemplated these partnerships while facing a future alone. The significance could not have been lost on her. I was more focused on Denise than on the others. Her stone face did not soften.

"For a while, many PALS [People with ALS] will want to be independent and accept no help," the woman running the seminar gently cautioned the new caregivers. They seemed so nervous. Denise leaned toward me from her chair. "That's me," she said in a thick whisper. "No help." I nodded. I know, I thought to myself, independent until the end.

Denise takes pride in proving herself independent and self-reliant. Fair enough. Doing for ourselves allows us to believe we are ahead of the game. Feeling that we are outpacing the Grim Reaper, despite what we know on another level, can keep us from sinking into despair and withdrawing from people around us.

Denise lives in fear of that inevitable day when cherished independence takes its place as a memory. So do I. But Denise ventures further. She goes out of her way to dispute the notion that she needs any assistance. In one conversation at her home, I suggested she might find a caregiver helpful. The woman bridled. "Why would I need a caregiver right now?" The edge in her voice cut clear.

"Maybe you would not feel so alone," I offered.

"Why would I feel alone? I have been divorced fifteen years. This is not new." She sounded very impatient. And defensive. "I am fine," she announced abruptly.

"And you really don't feel alone?"

"Why would I feel alone?" she repeated. For a moment, I thought she was going to come across the table at me. "I was alone before the disease happened. A caregiver is a caregiver, not a companion," she insisted. I nodded and said nothing. "A caregiver you pay to blow your nose and do whatever is necessary," she went on.

Denise sounded disparaging of such help. "I have hitched myself to friends I want to be around and who understand what I am going through." She stared at me fiercely. "They know the ups and downs of the disease." The companionship of friends, Denise claims, is all she needs and all she wants or will accept.

"Might you change your mind about opening the door to another person?" I asked.

"I would think that a man would not want to get attached to me now, knowing that I am going to die. Sooner or later, he would have to take care of me on a daily basis. I do not want that." Denise had been alone for many years. She knew little else. Her brief marriage and divorce had come years before sickness. She had been involved with someone, but he headed for the hills soon after hearing her diagnosis.

"People who have a spouse often feel worse because they consider themselves to be a burden." Denise paused and swallowed hard with emotion. "I don't have that worry. In a way, I feel I am more fortunate. This is my feeling about me. I am not here to make judgment calls about other PALS who are married and have kids. I never had kids, so I would not know what that is like in the first place."

Denise does not know the emotional fuel that flows from

a family. It was not clear if she wanted to know. Knowing leads to feeling, and that may be threatening because it pushes high emotion into your face. Novocain seemed to be the drug of choice for her.

If a bedrock belief in self and future possibilities burns within, it is fed and nurtured by those around us, people we love who love us. That must not be minimized. I know. Meredith and our kids traveled with me, walking across hot coals and through storms of emotional pain with me when cancer came twice. They paid a price and then offered me strength.

You confuse folks, Denise, I thought. You complain about a lack of emotional support but resent it when it is offered. So you drive people away. That was my snapshot of her, pushing others away and wondering why the people so important in her life were not there for her.

After months of insisting that she did not want me to write about her family, Denise turned in her tracks and arranged a dinner with them, an engagement she negotiated without consulting me. She wants to get me off her back, I figured. I suspected she would indulge me and break bread with her relatives, then revert to her former stance.

Denise's folks had driven in from the desert for a short visit before leaving for a cruise around Australia. They were staying with their other daughter, Lori, and her family. As we walked into the modern, spacious home in Calabasas, I warned Denise to be careful not to knock the chip off her shoulder as we passed through the doorway. She laughed.

The group sat there and eyed one another. The family was polite but reserved. They were sizing me up, sitting with their full weight on their very own Pandora's box.

I made eye contact with each, and they stared back and through me. They had to feel threatened by the very idea of Denise talking about them to a stranger. Denise had told me she does not speak about ALS with her family anymore.

After the hors d'oeuvres disappeared and the small talk trailed off, I turned to Denise's mother. "Denise tells me you make pot roast by cooking the meat in coffee instead of wine. Do you really do that?" I asked, looking appropriately dubious. Selma, Denise's mother, had been leaning back in the sofa, as if pulling back from a painful subject. I saw her relax a bit.

"You should try it," she said enthusiastically, grabbing on to this safe subject. "It is good. You'll like it." As we began to talk about Denise and this book, we steered clear of specifics. Others slowly joined the conversation.

The living room, with its high cathedral ceiling, lacked intimacy and warmth, both of which this dialogue badly needed. The tiptoeing seemed loud. Denise tried to bait the others a bit, but no one would bite.

Dinner wound down and the evening warmed. Denise's parents agreed to address any questions as they came to mind. Al and Selma seemed to believe me when I told them I wanted their takes on Denise and that I would listen. The couple could be reached by e-mail while on the cruise. Communicating electronically would be an interesting way to engage them, I figured, building in distance and retreating from in-your-face intimacy.

"Why didn't you ask them anything?" Denise demanded the minute we climbed back into her van. "Come on, Denise," I answered. "This was not the right moment. You did not let me meet these people until now. I was not going to attack them." Denise had not wanted me digging into family issues. Now she was throwing a shovel at me. "Besides," I added, "they are leaving tomorrow. Let it be on good terms, and let's keep the dialogue going." Denise said nothing.

Actually, I had enjoyed talking with the family, but for parents of a dying woman, they did seem disengaged from their daughter. My sense was that the distance grew out of their feeling pushed away, and that they were mystified by Denise's alienation from them. At the same time, I did wonder how they could merrily sail away when their younger daughter was so sick. We all are different.

My first e-mail to parts unknown was vague, asking only how the family was dealing with Denise's sickness. Selma and Al waited a few days. "I am still, I guess, in a state of denial," Selma's e-mail started. "It is difficult for a mother to come to grips with something like this and keep thinking that maybe there will be a cure or something to slow down the progression."

And from Al: "Our acquaintances are shocked and sympathetic upon learning about Denise. Most of our friends always inquire as to how she is getting along and are amazed at her attitude and fortitude in doing all the things she is doing instead of just resigning herself to the inevitable." I was taken aback. Why are you relaying the feelings of friends instead of your own?

These messages, Al's in particular, showed little emotion. What Al had to say read like a prepared statement. My concerns were about the family, not about unnamed acquaintances who might not even know Denise. Feelings did not seem to flow easily from this retired attorney or his wife.

When relations in a family are complex to begin with, a serious sickness can up the ante dramatically. Their issues must go way back, I thought.

Denise's sister, Lori, had worn discomfort on her face during our visit. In the next week, when I was back in New York, my phones messages went unreturned. Instinct said the obvious, that she was avoiding the prospect of painful questions and had no interest in serving up answers. Days went by, and then Lori's husband, Ron, an attorney outside Los Angeles, called, graciously agreeing to discuss Denise.

Ron, like Denise, had worked for Harry, the attorney who succumbed to ALS. It was Denise who had introduced Ron to Lori. I asked Ron if he believed this family conflict was about more than ALS. "It is dredging up old stuff, is my guess," he said. "I know that Denise's folks were pretty strict when they were growing up. Al was a workaholic and not around a lot of the time. Denise has anger about that." Ron stopped. "And the parents are not the warmest, touchy-feely people around. I could see that they might not give the kind of support she wanted."

Ron spoke carefully, choosing words slowly and suggesting that the family traveled a two-way street. "Denise is not the warmest person, either. They are cut from the same cloth, all friendly but not necessarily warm. A lot of Selma is in her. They are all very nice people, including Denise, but they are rigid and need to be in control. So Denise comes by it honestly."

"It is very difficult to approach her if you are perceived

to be critical," Ron continued. "Denise is very defensive. And she asks for nothing. I wonder: What does she want?" For me, this was not a new message, only a different messenger. Denise seemed to want others to reach out to her, I thought once again, so she could push them away.

As Denise and her family issues were swirling in my head, I was surprised to receive an e-mail from a care manager at the ALS Association in California. I had met her sometime before. This health care professional had served as Denise's caseworker and offered her own experience and take on Denise's mind-set.

"Maybe Denise translates a relationship as in some way losing some of her independence. She cannot tolerate feeling dependent or reliant on anyone else, including me. Sometimes I feel that she pushes her family away, too."

Reliance on imperfect people—is there a perfect family?—did not sit well with Denise. She had told me in numerous conversations that her parents were not there for her. Period. They did not care to know anything about ALS and thought only about themselves. Their communications to me said otherwise, but those communications were to me and not messages for her. Actions speak louder than e-mails.

The ALS care manager had it right. Denise cannot bear the prospect of depending on anyone. Allowing illness to send her back under her parents' wings may take on particular potency given the family's history. So Denise seems to cut loose the people around her and then bemoan the sad fact that they are not at her side.

In an e-mail to Selma, I asked how Denise's ALS had changed the family. Her reply: "At the time when Denise learned she had ALS she was going to a therapist who we felt was turning her hostile toward the whole family," Selma wrote. "Our family has always been close and concerned with one another's welfare but she resisted any attempts for anyone in the family to get close to her . . ."

Blaming a therapist for Denise's disengagement seemed defensive, and yet I could feel pain coming from Selma. "The family nevertheless continued to include Denise to the extent that she would let us," she continued. "We often wonder if Denise is angry with us that she became the victim of ALS. The thought also occurred that she feels we are genetically responsible. Denise's older sister, Lori, was diagnosed with lupus four years prior to Denise's diagnosis. Lori's reaction has been the opposite of Denise's and has brought her closer than ever within the family."

I found myself feeling bad for everyone. These people might well feel they were standing in Denise's corner. They also knew they were standing on trial. It was getting easier for me to understand why each of them felt as they did.

Denise may want strong support, but on her own terms. Her refusal to recognize the effort and emotion coming from her family is her way of coping. To Selma's credit, she expressed determination neither to judge Denise nor to give up.

"Although the whole family has been similarly rebuffed by Denise," Selma continued in her e-mail, "we have continued to do whatever she has permitted us to do to support her. We do not know if her asserted independence is to show us how strong she is or whether she is attempting to lessen the impact of what is inevitable.

"Our family would all like to be included with Denise, but since she chooses otherwise, we are willing to concede and are grateful that she is able to find the satisfaction and fulfillment that she is getting with the people and activities with which she is involved. Our family is resigned to doing what Denise will permit us to do, and are aware that we will be much more of a part of Denise's life in the hopefully distant future."

I forwarded Selma's e-mail to Denise, and the silence screamed. Then one dark morning this screed was waiting quietly on my computer: "N A I V E, N A I V E. First I started to cry out of anger and then I just shook my head and laughed. THEY DON'T GET IT!!! Even at this point. It's not about excluding them from anything or blame." Denise went on to enumerate her complaints about how manipulative her parents have long been in her life. She disputed their claims of wanting to be close.

Selma had written this: "Denise has resisted any attempts for anyone in the family to get close to her." Denise replied, "They DON'T know how to get close. Do you know that NO One has said to me, 'I'm sorry that you have this. I can't imagine how you feel.' They would be shocked as to my answer on this. This is how 'off' the charts they are . . . My parents couldn't even hold my hand, let alone sit next to me when the doctor read the diagnosis! They are on the sidelines because they wish to be."

Denise bristled as she told me in a follow-up phone call that her father, along with her siblings and in-laws, had adopted a paternalistic attitude toward her. "My brother-in-law Ron, brother Steve and Dad have powwows all the time about me—what is best for me, and then they pressure me to do what is best. Why aren't I INCLUDED in this powwow? Don't I have a say as to WHAT IS BEST for Denise?"

Denise had not displayed such anger before. "They—all of them—are NEVER going to change. It's still stupid Denise who never amounted to anything."

Self-esteem is not Denise's strong suit to begin with, and the pain of feeling like a second-class citizen in her own family precedes her illness. For her, as for many among us, illness has inflated to new proportions all that already existed .

The white heat of disease was melting the family glue, with pure anger the by-product. These are good people, which should make anyone wonder how common this kind of conflict is. Fighting in the family feels safer than taking on a dread disease. Fear and helplessness combine explosively. Old issues detonate at the most vulnerable moment. Chronic illness puts families under siege.

For me, this was a variation on a theme. I had pulled away from those closest to me when colon cancer piled on multiple sclerosis, and an unhealthy dose of self-absorption got the best of me. Maybe family becomes a safe house for pent-up rage.

The irony is that family feuds, whatever their makeup, are almost beside the point; fighting sickness remains a solitary battle. No matter how loving a family, however attentive a friend, in the end, we die alone, and in sickness, we live alone. No one can fully understand our ordeals. The challenges to each of us become highly personal. Cumulative weariness with the struggle whispers, and only we hear. No wonder our families feel threatened.

For the sick to complain bitterly to our families would be to drive away those dearest to us. So we shrink back and keep our silence. We see the burden we have become, though, often, no such heavy weight exists.

DENISE PULLED INTO the driveway and hit the automatic door opener at her ranch house off the Ventura freeway. It is a modest structure, a little drab on the exterior, but what the place lacks in charm is more than compensated for by convenience. Denise drove the van into her garage, within feet of an inside door leading directly into the kitchen.

The sparsely furnished interior make the place look like a way station. I had the strong impression that Denise had never moved in. She seemed to be camping out among computers and cartons. There was no sense of place, nor any sign of personal investment. There were no plants, no pets, and a refrigerator stocked with only bare essentials. The place reflected a one-day-at-a-time mentality. This is a temporary stop, I thought.

The house did seem a safe haven, though, and once inside, with the doors locked, Denise did seem secure. With her, I knew, there is no such thing. Weeks earlier, I had found an early-morning e-mail from her with an alarming, cryptic plea in the subject heading: "I fell. Call me." The rest of the e-mail was blank. I called Denise later that morning. She was upset, badly bruised, and rattled from the tumble.

Now, on her turf, she showed me the spot next to the garage where she had gone down hard. She had been taking out the garbage, carrying more than she could handle. The incident pointed up what I had already learned in my life.

Test the illusion of normalcy, and watch out. Anything can happen, anytime, anyplace. More to the point, Denise had been trying to do too much at one time and without backup.

"You are a loner, aren't you?" I asked.

"I spend about ninety per cent of my time by myself."

"And before you got sick?"

"Same." She was not about to change.

"What is wrong with holding a hand?" I wondered. "And wouldn't it have been easier with a family?"

"A spouse and kids?" she almost demanded. "No. I am alone in dealing with this." She paused to swallow. "And I am grateful. I do not feel guilty, avoiding compromising a spouse or children's lives by dealing with this and making them go through it." Another pause. "Because it is hell," she said. "It is hell."

She went on: "I cry when I see families of PALS because I know what they are going through." Denise had thought the issue through and was not making excuses. "I became very close with three girlfriends, Cathy, Shelley, and Cheryl, whose husbands, Andy, Ernie, and Jeff had ALS," she told me with emotion. "The families all had either young kids or older ones." Denise recounted their ordeals. "My girlfriends did not sleep at night for over a year because they were taking care of their husbands."

The men died within nine months of each other. Denise believes that her friends with ALS were the lucky ones. "I am happy for them, that they are relieved of the confinement in that cocoon of the body, and the inner soul is out and free. But their families have suffered so much. And for them, still it is not over."

"ALS is in a category by itself, isn't it?" I asked. Denise practically whispered the word "yes." There is a culture of death with this disease. "Yes, because there are no expectations of a long life," she answered quickly. "There is only the certainty of death. ALS offers nothing except the knowledge that you better live your dreams pretty quickly."

By now in the conversation my own self-absorption was kicking in. I was trying to determine for myself whether I, under any circumstances, could stop thinking about that last hideous state, the loss of all control and certain death. How does a person keep going?

For those of us with our own different diseases, the scenario strikes the classic chord, that someone always has it worse than you. The question —"How does she just go on?" —rumbled around my head in the middle of the night, and I got out of bed to e-mail her.

"It is not easy," her e-mailed answer began. "I wake up thinking 'Am I going to fall today? Is there going to be a physical change for the worse?' Then I think about what fun things there are for me to do now and in the future. This gives me enjoyment, a purpose, and keeps my mind working. It helps keep the depression at a lower level."

"Do you ever think about your end," I asked her in a subsequent phone call. There was a silence, then a soft moan. "Yeah. I sometimes go there. The thought of dying from ALS is not frightening."

"It's not?"

"No. How much will I be able to endure? That is the question." And by the time you answer that, I thought, it will be too late to do anything about it. You will be paralyzed and a prisoner of a moribund body.

"You never get over having the disease," Denise said softly. "This will let up the day I am free from ALS, and that will be when I am dead." We were sitting outdoors in the sunshine at an overpriced California fruit and smoothie stand. Denise's remark came without self-pity or any other agenda. "I have seen too many friends progress. I know what is ahead of me."

"Five years in, you have to be a different person."

"You bet."

"Are you a better person?"

"I am far more compassionate, far more loving and happier, even though I've been told, 'You are going to die and there is nothing we can do.'" ALS had opened up a positive piece of this woman. How ironic to be reborn and die from the same disease.

Identity and illness have fused. ALS has given life a meaning Denise could not find another way. It is, she says, a gift. "If I did not have ALS, I never would have met the most wonderful people in my life. I have friends who are so good. They keep me going."

She has replaced family, flesh and blood, with the ALS community, those with the misfortune to be like her, along with their families and friends. They may have but one thing in common, but these people have become boon travel companions, generous and helpful. For Denise, ever independent, it has been a revelation.

When she moved to the Ventura place, she needed help. "It was the first time in my life I asked," she said. "And to have twenty-five or thirty people, almost all from the ALS community, come and help me, well, I did not know that many people who could be my friends before I was diagnosed," she said in a wobbly voice but with a look of resolve on her face. "So I am blessed to have these people in my life."

For all her widening circle, Denise remains wary. When she takes from friends, occasionally leaning harder than she can tolerate, she pushes back, retreating into herself. The risks are too great. She is still a loner.

DENISE SEEMED MORE open than usual one sunny day in California. "I was an unhappy person before I was diagnosed with ALS. I had no life. There was no fun. No traveling. Just work." And now? "I have a disease and I am living a new life. I've been given a chance for a second life out of that life."

What she found was the formula for dying, which happens to be the same as a plan for living. "I say, 'You need to appreciate every day. Do something for you. Light a candle. Go outside. Smell the fresh air.'" She looked radiant in her up moments.

"I am living a life I did not live for forty-eight years," she went on. "Now I am cramming it in. I am a new me." One of the linchpins of her new life is advocacy work. She speaks to high school classes and has made a video that was delivered to elected officials in Washington. "I have found my purpose in life. Getting the word out helps me through each day."

When Denise got her diagnosis in 2001, she had immediately focused on trips she wanted to take, experiences she needed to have. Then she wilted, falling into a deep depression. "I got into these funks where I locked myself in my house for four or five days," she recalled.

For eight months, she wallowed and wailed and demanded to know, "Why me?" "I was incredibly depressed and did not know how to deal with my feelings and how to go forward." She was medicated that first year. "You have to be," she said. And she spent hours with a therapist. Finally, the therapist got through. "'What happened to your goals, who you wanted to be?'" Denise remembered her demanding.

At that moment an advocate's identity was born. "I got very active with the ALS Association, and it turned my life around, my meeting other PALS and helping them with their lives." She finally decided to "accept and move on."

"Are you really learning to accept?"

"People fight accepting ALS, but as years go on, we begin learning to accept. What good is fighting the inevitable? That does not clear a path to the next step of your life."

"Which is?"

"Dying."

The struggle for any ALS patent is to stay up. Down was where Denise found herself on a December Saturday, sitting on a suitcase at JFK watching cars scream by. She was cooling her heals in the freezing temperature, waiting for Meredith and me, and not at all happy about having to sit. She was arriving in snowy New York only weeks before Christmas.

Denise was good company but could not allow herself to be simply a guest. The role did not suit her. She insisted on cooking and cleaning, as if those were a payback or there were a point to be made. And for her, there was. These small issues were all about control.

A cold wind blew, and a patchwork of drifts decorated our property during Denise's last days with us. On the final day, a blizzard threatened. I walked out of our bedroom to find a bulging suitcase in the hall by the guest room. I could hear Denise fussing.

She had decided to abandon ship a day early, hoping to avoid the snow. There had been no collaboration, no discussion, not a mention of switching gears. The woman was up and ready to roll. Her airline ticket had already been adjusted in the predawn hours.

"Please help Denise with her suitcases," I yelled to the boys as they were grabbing their own backpacks and books.

"No," Denise's voice rang out sharply through the house. "No," she repeated. "I can carry my own things."

"I am sure you can," I said to her, "but the boys are big and strong, and it will be good for them." Denise simply ignored me as she brushed by. I stared silently at her back.

Later, in an e-mail, she elaborated on her need to keep up her appearance and, of course, control: "My pride and image are in the work I do now or did then. How I look is important to me. That is control. Being organized and trying to make it perfect through my eyes, that is me. But I've noticed with the disease progressing that the more independence and control I lose with my body, I now see myself trying to control everything else in my life. I feel losing independence and accelerating control go hand-in-hand."

Bingo—though a difficult admission. Low self-esteem had long since created the control issue, for, as she said, when she was in charge, she felt like somebody. Then throw in ALS. "When you are dealt a blow like this, you are out of control. You do not have control of your body. So I control other things that I know I can control, just anything. I always take the lead, in anything I do. Have you noticed?"

I nodded and kept my mouth shut. "It just happens. I try not to take over. I know now what I'm doing, so I try not to do it." Whatever Denise's pattern of manufacturing control, ALS had upped the stakes in her struggle for ownership of anyone's most prized possession: self.

"Something or someone else is going to have control over my body. It will not be me anymore. I know that, and it is scary. As I keep saying, how far do I want to go with this disease? How long will I let someone take care of me?" A page was turning. Circling the subject was as close as I had gotten to the idea of suicide. Denise's face became granite whenever this topic reared up.

"We need to talk about that, sooner or later," I said to Denise. "Your hints take us only so far. What is your worst-case scenario about losing control?"

"That I will not be able to care for myself," she answered, "to take a shower by myself. I will not be able to blow my own nose. Scratch an itch. Those are the ultimate control issues," she said forcefully, "because if I lose control and someone else has to do it, I have to ask for everything."

She could not live with that. "No," she quickly responded. "Then caretakers are in control of my body. I don't want caretakers to think they know what's best for me without asking me."

"You said you will be mentally intact," I pointed out.

"You also will be physically dependent. Exactly where does that leave you?"

"Everything comes down to how much I can endure."

"You have said that more than once. Please take me further in your thinking."

"I just feel people have the right to choose what they want to do with their lives." She paused. "Where they go and when they leave are very personal decisions."

"In Mitch Albom's *Tuesdays with Morrie,* physical helplessness overtook Morrie. He suffered a total loss of privacy, lost control of his body, had a nurse wiping his butt," I said. "Isn't that where you are headed?"

"Physically, yeah. Do I want that kind of life? It's a decision I will face." She hung back, not about to sign on any dotted line. "Do I want to prolong my life? I have a choice in whether or not I want to have a feeding tube, if I want to be on oxygen, if I want a ventilator. Those are the main ways of living longer with ALS."

"And?"

Denise just stared into my eyes.

As the body fails, control and the last word still belong to the patient. Maintaining that power becomes the lingering uncertainty. "Absolutely." Denise's tone was urgent.

"Can you assume that nobody will step in and overrule you?"

"There are documents I will be drawing up that will say what I want and what I don't."

A year passed before we returned to the topic. During a phone call, I raised the subject again. What gives?

"The document is almost finished. It spells out what I want. It is called an Advanced Directive." The papers

detailed what, if any, heroic measures were acceptable.
"Right. Everyone should have one. Do you?" Don't change
the subject, Denise.

The document, of course, said nothing about Denise
taking matters into her own hands. "Right," she said
softly. "Look, I have that right. I am over eighteen. It is my
body, not theirs. It is not what they want. It's what I want.
Ending your life your own way is your business." Denise
did not budge or reveal herself.

"You keep referring to 'they.' Who would 'they' be?"

Her response backed off the reference to "they." "I was
bitter and very angry with my family," she wrote by way
of explanation. "I've now accepted them for what they are
and cannot change them."

I doubted her new placid attitude toward her family.
Her relationship with her parents and siblings had gnawed
at her for so long. But Denise seemed to be done with the
subject.

The family might be invited in as players when things
got bad, I suggested. "Do they know your wishes?"

"No. No one does."

"Would your family try to overrule you?"

"I don't know. I never asked them." The inevitabilities
are clear. "They know that I'm going to die from this." She
paused. "And I think they know what is going to happen
between now and then."

Denise owed me nothing, including private information.
There was no reason to assume she would share her plan.
"Have you thought about taking your own life?" I asked
directly. The question was blunt, though not out of line. We
had discussed options without explicitly defining them.

"Have I considered suicide? Oh yes, in the beginning," she said, looking at me.

"Where do you come down on it these days?"

She paused. "I decided, no."

"No, you have not decided?"

"No, I am not going to do it. I have way too much advocacy work to do." I knew this answer was today's special. "We will see," she said. By now, this line of conversation had stretched across the continent, not to mention the years, during visits, on the phone and in e-mails. I assume you would need to plan how to do anything yourself or get someone to help. We sat in silence, looking at each other. "I agree." That was it.

"That is all you are going to say about it, isn't it?"

Denise laughed. "I have a folder with all kinds of information and I am not ready to open that door."

"I am not trying to put ideas in your head," I told her. "I am only asking if that ultimate act is what you have been alluding to in our many conversations."

"It is a thought every PALS has," she allowed. "I mean, who the hell wants to go down the ALS road?"

"You have the power to do what you want."

"Yes," she said quickly. "And hurrah for Oregon," she shouted, an obvious reference to the only state to legalize physician-assisted suicide.

ALS complicates an already complicated subject. "If communication is not available, and there is only silence, no one can know what you want or what you may wish you had done," Denise added. Passing the point of no return would give me nightmares. "In the very last stages of ALS, you are in lockdown," she pointed out again. "Then you need a plan." But she insisted that, so far, there was no exit strategy.

"This will be like getting my walker," she said. "I hated the walker idea. Hated it." She was having trouble getting the words out. "Then the time came. I decided to get it." And? "Now, it is good. I am taking it as it comes."

"Ending it all," I said, "of course, is different."

"Yes."

In show business, timing is everything. The risk of Denise finding herself incapable of action hangs over her. "There always are ways. If it is past that point, there are things I can do." She paused. "I am not going to get into it in any detail."

ON A WARM late autumn Saturday afternoon a few years ago, Denise and I snaked through California mountain passes, heading home from a drive along the ocean. The wind was up. The Pacific had been rough. The terrain inland was sharp and craggy. A feeling of proximity to the elements that I do not get in the middle of New York City was not lost on me.

Denise said suddenly, "I want to show you one more thing."

"Go for it," I answered.

We drove a while longer, listening to the wind and taking in the terrain. "It is the pet cemetery where my kitties are buried," she offered. "The place is so peaceful and very beautiful," she added. "I feel so calm when I am there."

Denise had talked repeatedly about her beloved pets in our many conversations. In fact, her cats seemed to be the only living things she held dear. "I have never loved anything more in my life," she declared more than once. I found it difficult to relate to her intensity of connection. I had asked if the love she received from her animals was greater than what she had felt from any person in her life. "Absolutely!!!" came an emphatic reply.

In truth, her pets were her family. "The kitties were my everything. I never had kids, so the cats were my children. There was not anything I would not do for them to make them happy and comfortable."

The deaths of those animals, it seemed, would fore-shadow her own. "Crystal died just six days before my diagnosis. Worst week in my entire life, experiencing the death of something I've loved so much and then hearing of my diagnosis."

Denise took out a tissue. "I thought, immediately, if I die before Stained, who would take such good care of her? Part of me died that week. Stained felt my pain and was there with her comforting ways. I was closer to her than ever. She lived another two and a half years, and I was home with her. I knew she would die soon, so I cherished every day I was with her."

"Did Stained teach you anything about living or dying?" I asked. I could hear a soft sound and turned, realizing she was weeping. "Denise, are you okay?" Again, nothing. "I will e-mail you later," she said in a tiny, halting voice.

"Okay," the e-mail would read when I was back in New York. "I have stopped crying. My cats comforted me in ways humans could not. Call me back. I am having a tough time answering that question." I waited and called. "I am sorry," she said. "I was thinking about everything. My kitties taught me the power of love. That's all."

She could not bear to cremate the cats when the time came, instead burying each in a tiny casket. As we sat in that pet cemetery on that peaceful afternoon, our conversation took a predictable turn. Denise turned to me and announced out of nowhere that after she died, she intended to be cremated.

"Where do you want your ashes to go?" I asked, expecting her to talk about her spot high above the Pacific. She sat in silence and turned the car back on.

"Pacific Palisades?" I guessed.

She did not move, then looked up one last time, swinging around to see her kitties' graves. For a moment, the tiny woman seemed focused. I stared into her eyes. Perhaps we were home. Denise said nothing. Then we drove away.

....

Reflections

Choosing the Way to Live

When the end is in sight, the choices in our lives become telling, defining who we are and what really matters to us. Denise understands the reality that we die alone. She forces us to accept that each of us concocts a different formula for getting by as we grapple with serious illness. For some, maintaining a large community to offer support becomes important. Surrounding ourselves with other people offers solace. For me, reaching for the safety and warmth of family and friends has always been instinctive. For

Denise, the search for solitude, a self-imposed isolation, is the modus operandi.

Many of us may see this as a way of hiding most appropriate for those who cannot bear to engage others. We judge isolation as wrong and emotional distance as cold. The sick, especially those close to dying, are supposed to be dependent and almost apologetic for their condition. They are expected to compensate for their abnormal state by being nice and deferential, grateful for any helping hand, welcoming of anyone who offers intimacy to one so broken.

Denise's approach to her illness and a death not far down the road is anything but deferential. She requires independence without compromise, then resents being alone. She refuses to lean on others but does so with a stiff arm and an unspoken demand. In the few instances where she does reveal her neediness, she expresses anger at that need. This is a painful cycle. And while I worked hard to create a keep-your-distance intimacy between us, it was hard won. I simply could not identify with her method of coping, and it left me deeply confused.

Was I as rigid as she in my insistence that she be close on my terms? Aren't we all at times trapped by our own rigidity? The sick should not have to be different. Or perhaps, they should be given greater leeway for forging their own path, frustrating though it may be for the rest of us.

We all require a level of patience that is in short supply in our busy lives. Being a friend to a mortally injured comrade is a commitment that takes time and levels of acceptance we may not have previously known. It is easy to decide that the Denises of the world are beyond caring because they seem to stand back from others.

A lasting image of Denise says otherwise. At a candle-light vigil in Washington, D.C., for the ALS fallen, Denise wept silently as she struggled to hold four flickering candles and repeated the names of lost friends over and over in a hoarse whisper. Clearly, I thought, this lady cares deeply. She reached out to the dead that night. Maybe her unwillingness to turn to the living says more about us than her.

three

Buzz Bay

Keeping the Faith

"I AM OKAY," Buzz Bay said in a shaky voice, blinking away sleep and grinning up at me. The forty-six-year-old man in the bed was gaunt and hairless, the pale portrait of cancer that so many among us sadly see in our own worlds. He had been admitted a day earlier to a hospital in Beach Grove, Indiana, with a ureter painfully blocked by pressure from a malignant tumor.

A white hospital gown was opened at the side a crack, displaying tubes growing from strange places on his body, stretching into various bottles and containers attached to a pole on wheels. The urine output of one kidney trickled out of his body through a rubbery hose he wore out his side.

Buzz had just awakened from a gentle doze, and he was instantly ready to talk. "How was your flight out here?" he asked. "Did you find the hospital easily enough?"

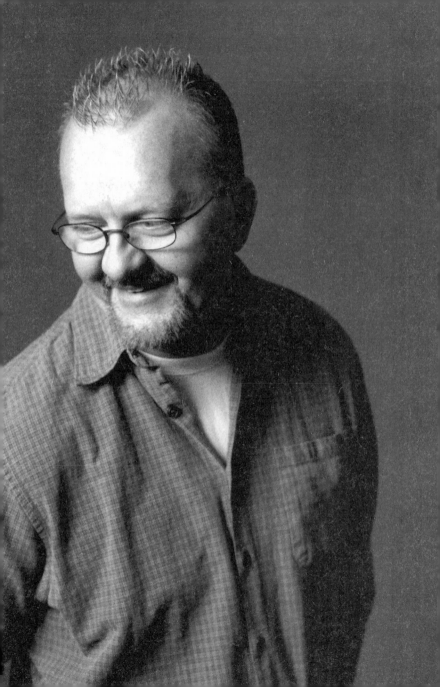

"Buzz," I asked back, "how are you feeling?"

"Oh, I am fine."

"Really?"

"Yup. Upright and taking nourishment," he answered, hardly upright at all. This was not the first time nor would it be the last, that Buzz kissed off that question. As with Denise, a long warm-up had preceded the visit. We had talked numerous times on the phone and exchanged e-mails—words, not intimacy, at a safe distance.

This was not the way I had planned our first meeting. I had been about to head for Indiana to teach at DePauw University when I received a call from The Leukemia & Lymphoma Society, telling me Buzz was in the hospital.

Soon enough, I found myself in Indianapolis, speeding south from the airport with my friend from DePauw. We cruised down the interstate, a straight shot of concrete, into the heartland. I was worried. In our recent telephone conversations, the incoming chatter had been weak and without energy, betraying the unmistakable sound of a weary man. Buzz had been in the middle of a chemotherapy cycle, the treatments exacting a terrible toll.

Buzz has non-Hodgkin's lymphoma. Lymphomas are cancers that grow in the lymphatic system, an integral part of the body's immune defense system. As with most cancers, lymphomas take many forms. One type, Hodgkin's disease, can be relatively benign, with survival rates exceeding 90 percent.

Non-Hodgkin's, though, is an aggressive and virulent lymphoma. It can be treated but not cured. The chance of surviving five years with the disease is less than 50 percent. This brand of lymphoma struck down activist Dick

Gregory, King Hussein of Jordan, and Jacqueline Kennedy Onassis.

Still, Buzz has always been curiously upbeat, with depleted strength but an expansive optimism that flies in the face of the facts. I was unsure about meeting him for the first time at his worst, but he encouraged my visit, particularly since I was going to be in the area. Plus, our brief encounter would allow me to meet not just the man but the family. We would all use the next few hours to size up each other.

I was the complete stranger from out there somewhere, a cultural Martian in Buzz's world. The west side of Manhattan and the rural climbs of southern Indiana are very different lands. Each of us needed the comfort level I had sought and eventually found with Denise. Building that kind of trusting relationship meant bridging a wide gap.

I watched Buzz and watched him watching me. "I like your outfit," he said, referring to my blue jeans and a sweatshirt featuring a duck. Susan, Buzz's wife, sat beside him in the small waiting room. We had slowly walked down the long corridor away from his room and roommate in search of privacy. Their son, Ryan, nine years old at the time, sat ducking the conversation, reading and fidgeting, seemingly oblivious to the stranger in their midst.

Buzz seemed remarkably at ease but studied in his responses. He showed a natural talent for deflection, steering the talk away from himself. When are you getting out of here? "I don't know. When are you leaving town?" Are you okay? "I am here."

Though clearly in pain and exhausted, he seemed oddly

detached from his illness. I had noticed this already. Our deal from the beginning was that he was going to open up about coping with cancer and joining the army of survivors struggling with chronic conditions. Our e-mails and telephone conversations had become routine, however. We were not grappling with the ever present issues of illness, and little of substance had been said. Now here I was, in his face and ready to put the Ping-Pong paddles away.

Buzz looked at me as if deciding his next move. Maybe he was surprised that I had actually shown up, carrying a tape recorder at that. This was sudden and serious, and he seemed not quite ready to let the games begin.

This hairless man had an easy way about him. He seemed to like people, if not what came from their mouths. He was guarded, defended, a shrink might say. His winces were subtle and slight as the questions began. His patter did not vary. Talking face-to-face at last, making eye contact, may have seemed threatening. I felt the awkwardness of the moment, too.

Buzz seemed determined to appear confident or at least comfortable with his physical condition. He clearly was exhausted and in pain, surrounded by a family that seemed bewildered. But there he sat, dispensing limitless cheer. Throughout the afternoon, the guy smiled and quipped and never seemed to walk off the stage. He was playing to the audience. Me. The jokes were the giveaway.

"How are you?"

"I woke up this morning. That's good."

He had his routines down. Even as Rome was burning, Buzz was playing the fiddle. Buzz, I would learn, is a naturally sunny and optimistic fellow. His glass is forever half-full. I do not want this to happen, the emotional reasoning goes, so happening it is not.

The ring is familiar. Dependable denial had formed the architecture of emotional survival for me, too. My denial was rooted in pushing away realities I could not bring myself to embrace. I could dance the two-step, revising any prognosis with the best of them. Denial kept me going. That talent can be a strong ally, a healthy coping mechanism, depending on how smartly it is applied.

If denial kept Buzz from clear and sensible thinking, that would be quite different. It was too soon to know, but the bright outlook seemed to be out of context, if not out of touch.

Beyond the quips, Buzz did make one fact, perhaps the most far-reaching about his life, strikingly clear. "I have a belief in God, a trust in my heart." He was going on the record. "You cannot see faith, but it is there," he said. "Our lives are built on that faith, and someday, our faith will take us to another level," he told me as I left the hospital. That belief system is stitched on every sleeve in Buzz's modest closet, even on his stained hospital gown.

A devout Christian, Buzz has beliefs that are ironclad and unshakable. "One way or another, I will be cured," Buzz would assure me repeatedly, "here on earth or in heaven."

That single assertion said it all. The faith game was new to me. Alien. But I was committed to listening.

FOUR MONTHS AFTER our accidental visit, a more ambitious itinerary and focused plan carried me back to Franklin, Indiana, the town where Buzz grew up and now lives with his family. Franklin is a small island in a sea of corn and soybeans, sitting twenty-five miles south of Indianapolis. The town is home to twenty-five thousand residents. There is an eerie order to the place. Houses are well kept and neat, the lawns manicured, the streets quiet and clean, really clean.

For a New Yorker, a small town in the Midwest was unfamiliar territory. Franklin was out of a coffee table book. The folks are mostly white, and they all seem to be smiling. There are churches on every block, planted and sprouting up next to each other like crops. This was 1950 in the new millennium. The Cleavers could have lived here.

The Bay home, an 1890s wood-frame farmhouse outside town, sits on a small road at the end of a crooked dirt path. There is a warm, homey feel to the old place. Odds and ends of a family's life—toys and shoes, books and magazines, stuff—lay on the floor in every part of each room. Buzz, Susan, and I settled into comfortable worn furniture.

Buzz appeared to be much improved from the hospital, his furnace rekindled. The tube draining his kidney had been removed two months earlier, after a scan indicated that the tumor blocking the flow of urine had shifted away. The painful pressure on his ureter was gone.

He seemed to have recovered, albeit temporarily, from the siege suffered during my first visit. He was a new person. He seemed relaxed, had put on weight and grown a head of hair. He was even more confident and cheerful than before.

Still, my "Hi, how are you?" was met with a smile and "Upright and taking nourishment." New man, old material.

An easterner's caricature of the Man from Main Street, Buzz appears to have stepped right out of a Jimmy Stewart movie, the straightforward standup guy utterly without guile, no rough edges. I kept prodding and poking, teasing and testing to see what he was concealing behind the smile. But the smile never disappeared.

Buzz and Susan have been married for twenty-five years. An attractive woman with an open face, this straightforward lady has a comfortable air about her. When Buzz went into his routines, she patiently chuckled and sighed with affection, almost rolling her eyes.

"You know Buzz," she would say, a common phrase in their circle of friends. Susan makes the family train run on time. She exhibits an understated resilience and is there for Buzz, without folding her identity into his. Just like Meredith, she can take a step away and call her husband on how he deals with his emotional health.

The two had met in junior high and were a couple through high school. Buzz went on to attend Johnson Bible College in Tennessee, while Susan studied nursing in Indiana. They were married in 1982. "Susan was the only one who would put up with me," Buzz said, laughing. "I always knew she would be my wife."

The couple adopted Ryan in 1995, after years of attempting to start a family. Buzz approaches parenting with the energy and enthusiasm of an adult who feels just plain lucky to have a child. The Bays are an inseparable threesome. Whither thou goest, they go together.

Buzz and I were getting serious when he remembered he needed to run a quick errand. We drove into town and circled the square, looking for a parking spot. What would take an hour in Manhattan took only a minute. Buzz was in better humor than I, as he walked and I stumbled down the street on this morning. He nodded to and greeted everyone we passed as if he recently had been elected mayor.

At my urging, Buzz cheerfully began describing his journey into illness, a tacky tale of missteps and miscues by his doctors. This had not been medicine in its finest hour. Buzz is a generous man, a true Christian who lives it as he sings it on Sundays. His equanimity did not crack as the story unfolded.

His journey into the medical maze began with a nagging case of athlete's foot, one that simply would not go away. "I am not an athlete. I tried different medicines and ointments, and it just kept getting worse." He laughed as he told me these facts, as if they were funnier than far-reaching. His voice did turn tense, though, as he continued.

"Then my family doctor said, 'There is a new medicine I want you to try, but I need you to take liver tests to make sure you can take it, because this medicine is very strong.'" The blood work came back with ambiguous and troubling results. An ultrasound, done at the same time to determine if the liver was enlarged for any reason, showed shadowing around the organ. That was not a good sign."

For Buzz, this all sounded routine. No one chose to suggest otherwise. Amazing, I thought. Is "paternalistic" a more accurate word? When colon cancer had come my way and tests got goofy, I was told what was happening in painful detail. Most doctors long ago stopped turning lights off on patients.

"Everyone in the office knew that something seemed

wrong but us," Buzz remembered. "The entire staff in the ER where this was done had seen the results. They knew the story and, besides, they knew Susan well. She works as a secretary in the emergency room at the hospital. That is where all this was being done, so we knew everyone."

This sounded like a conspiracy of silence. "Well, the privacy laws forbid unauthorized disclosures by medical people," Buzz said.

"Come on, Buzz," I said back. "These were your friends. They could have said something indirectly or sent a signal, grabbed an imaginary noose around their necks or whatever without breaking the law."

"Maybe they thought I already knew," Buzz suggested, turning the other cheek. "They asked me to take a CT scan." Still, Buzz saw no evil and asked no questions. "They made it sound like, no big thing. You are over forty. We just want to check things out." Buzz just did what he was told. "I thought, well, okay, I guess this must be no big thing." To anyone else, of course, a CT scan suggests that something might be very wrong. Doctors let Buzz think otherwise.

The scan was done. Doctors saw a mass on the screen. "'You know, this could be nothing,' the guy told me. 'Men over forty sometimes get these benign masses and they go away, and sometimes they are nothing at all. So don't let it worry you.'" That it actually could be something never entered his mind.

For me, suspicion starts with the word "sometimes," especially when uttered by a doctor. That word is a communications cop-out. "The doctor just did not want to worry us until there was something to worry about," Buzz said. Right.

The CT scan was rushed to Indiana University Medical Center. Specialists immediately reported back to the local doctor that the scan had determined the mass was malignant. Now there was something to worry about. Buzz still was told nothing. "Well, see, there was a mix-up at the doctor's office, and no one told us."

The cone of silence had dropped over the Bays. "The doctors were supposed to call us in and explain everything." Instead, "They just asked, 'Can you come in tomorrow? We want to do another scan of the mass, this time with a needle biopsy.'" Buzz did not know why the doctor wanted to repeat the procedure, and the doc was not talking.

Buzz ducked into a shop, and we headed home. He was making small talk again and staying on safe ground. He made tea. We sat around the kitchen table with Susan, who picked up the story. "We said to each other, 'This is kind of strange,'" she said, "but no one ever explained anything to us."

I could only wonder why Buzz and Susan were not running down the corridors by then, screaming for information at the top of their lungs. If an impending procedure seems "kind of strange," isn't it time to start asking why?

"Cancer was not even in my mind. I did not think anything about it," Buzz said again. Please, Buzz. "Look," he said gently, "I had such peace in my life. I just was not worried about it. I was very laid back." Got it, I thought. We do live on different planets. Peace is one thing, a blind eye to the truck bearing down on you is quite another.

Susan, who had studied nursing, might have known better. Opting for ignorance over information seemed so odd. Maybe this was homegrown emotional pain management. Doctors routinely prescribe strong medications for searing physical pain. We are grateful for that numbness, however temporary. Even short-lived denial can provide the same kind of palliative care, blunting emotional pain. Physician-assisted denial is legal and seemed to have been at work here.

Finally, Susan did open her eyes and realized there were blinking red lights in her face. "Something is not right here," she said to herself. Buzz caught the vibe. "I could tell she thought something was wrong." The subtle sense that something was amiss came less from the quality of the information than from the faces and body language of friends and colleagues. The sunshine had vanished.

"When we went in to the X-ray department, the whole mood had changed," Buzz continued. "No one would talk to us. Everybody was really aloof. They put us in this room by ourselves, which they had never done before. My sixth sense told me something was not kosher." Buzz still had not assumed the worst.

"It was the looks on their faces," Susan recalled. "I knew these people. Something was really wrong." Then she laughed softly and dug herself in deeper. "When we saw pictures from the first scan, you are not going to believe this," she said.

"What?" I pressed.

"We thought the mass was an extra kidney."

Even when danger is sensed, there can be pockets of adamant disbelief. Buzz's denial must have been contagious.

All came clear as Buzz was being prepped for a needle biopsy, a painful stab in the belly performed under a scan to guide the needle. The radiologist entered the room and asked if their family physician had talked to them. "I said 'no,'" Buzz remembered. "'I have not heard from anybody.'" There was a moment of silence. "The doctor realized we had no clue, and I will never forget the blank look on his face."

The doctor stood, staring at the Bays. "'You have no idea what you're facing, do you?'" Buzz recalled him saying. Buzz was bewildered. A moment passed. "'What you have is non-Hodgkin's lymphoma, and you have a malignant tumor in your belly,' the doctor said."

This moment of truth came on August 11, 2001, at eleven o'clock on a sunny Indiana morning. Buzz thought the scene was strange. "Funny" was the word he used to describe the moment. He also thought it strange that the memory was cemented into his mind. Odd would be if that recollection faded with time.

Buzz had talked before about the loneliness of illness, which I have decided for myself is unavoidable. The feeling of emotional abandonment by physicians, the very people who should be counselors as well as care providers, can be devastating. When that happens, a rapidly increasing sense of isolation is inevitable. I asked Buzz if he felt that. "I am afraid so," he answered. "I felt that Susan and I were left there to figure things out for ourselves."

Emotions came quickly. "My wife started crying. It was like I heard just sobs." Buzz stopped talking for a moment. "It was that weird moment. You hear it, but you really do not believe it. I said to the doctor, 'You said what? How can athlete's foot turn into cancer? I do not understand.' I was stunned."

"What else did you feel?" I asked.

Buzz had his answer at the ready. "Then I figured that when you are given lemons," he said with that smile, "you make lemonade." Great, I thought.

"That's it?"

Buzz only shrugged. A reality sandwich and a chaser of lemonade. Buzz had turned the other cheek so far he had performed a three-sixty.

Buzz was characteristically charitable, not angry, just quietly disappointed with the way he was treated by his doctors. He laughed self-consciously, ready to change the subject and move on.

"We were going into this completely blind" was his low-key complaint when I would not switch subjects.

"Did you say anything to the doctor?" I pressed.

"I said, 'This was a monumental crisis and decisions that we were going to be facing here, and not even to be told . . .'" Buzz responded, trailing off. "'Well, it just slipped through the cracks', is about all he said. 'That is a big crack to fill there, buddy,'" Buzz had answered.

"You sound as if you do not like doctors very much, Buzz." *legitimize*

"It's hard when they do not respect you," he allowed. His reliance on physicians might have tempered his willingness to blow his cool.

"Buzz, do you get angry at anything?" I asked. I could read the sincerity in his expression.

"Sometimes I do hurt" was all he would say.

We have no concept of what to expect when illness

comes. Vulnerability seeps from our bodies like a slow bleed. The quality of our connection to a trusted physician becomes an emotional lifeline. We lean at different angles and with varying degrees of force in our search for support.

When our heroes in white falter beneath our weight, we struggle to stay standing. Asked if the way he was handled by the doctors just added unnecessary emotional pain, Buzz looked at me as if that was about the stupidest question he had been asked. "Yes," he said with no embellishment.

WHEN PEOPLE HEAR the bad news, their reactions are as distinct as their personalities. Buzz's first reaction was shock, followed immediately by a joke. But in time, his attention shifted to others. "My caring instincts took over, and I just wanted to make sure my family and everybody was okay." For him, family and close friends, had to come first. Thoughts for himself and fear of the future were not on his radar screen.

Then he paid a visit to his church. "My minister told me to stop and allow what the doctor told me to sink in. 'What you do and feel at this moment will be your witness for the rest of your life,' he said. So I asked to be left alone for a minute."

Only one minute to contemplate and plan the rest of his life? "Not really a minute," he answered. "I was alone for a while. I needed to get myself together, to think. I prayed. I was asking God for help." He took a long breath. "I said, 'We will be in this together.'"

I wondered what Buzz thought his minister meant by

What you do and feel at this moment will be your witness. "He was telling me that how I present myself to other people in this moment of crisis, what I do with it, will define me."

"And are you at peace with that?" I asked.

"Yes. I am not a negative person. In fact, I think I stay pretty positive." This may explain his concern for others around him, even his cheerful face for all to see. If Buzz believes that at the end of the day he will be judged by the quality of how he handles his disease and perhaps death, his path is clearly marked.

I, too, have known the quest for grace in the face of sickness. The prospect of death for me remains distant, and my search has been secular. As far as I know, God has not chosen to hang out in my room. I can hear Buzz now, smiling and telling me, "Yes, He was there."

When I learned that I had multiple sclerosis and later cancer, there was a cacophony of silence in my head: the sound of nothing. One doctor suggested that my emotions ran the gamut from *a* to *b*. I am still listening for the telltale sounds of high emotion.

Buzz seems not to indulge in such emotion, either. Conduct in the face of illness is an intensely private negotiation with self. Going forth with grace is important to both of us. Buzz attaches a different meaning to grace. "God's grace is his magnificent, overwhelming love. Grace covers us."

In my world, grace goes in another direction, defined by an individual's conduct. Grace becomes doing right by others, those we care most about. Grace is my gift to them.

Grace means doing it well. A graceful exit, for example, means giving the journey your best moves.

Buzz also gives to others, in far greater quantity than he gives to himself. For him, assisting the next guy comes at the expense of his own emotional needs. The two are not mutually exclusive. I have experienced pain and suffering from illness and sought to find my way across myriad quality-of-life issues. I love my family, and want to comfort them. I believe that I give to others but I also want to take care of myself.

Fasten your mask first, the flight attendant advises grown-ups. Then take care of any children. Survive so that you can assist others. Threatening illness demands a period of self-absorption so that, afterward, we can help those we care about. Buzz was busy conspiring with the Lord, trying to figure out how to tend to the needs of everyone else. The mission of a devout Christian was well defined for him. He did not question what he had to do.

Buzz's moments alone on that day of reckoning produced this plea: "I asked God to make me, with whatever time I have, be a strong witness for him. Allow me to give other people hope when there seems to be no hope." He went on, as if preaching. "Help me to be strong for Susan and Ryan and just try to be the best husband and father that I can be." Finally, he added: "Help us as a family to fight with all that we have against this, and know that we did the best we could."

That was the first call to arms I had heard from Buzz. And then he tacked this on: "And allow our family to help other families to know that God is there no matter what."

He paused. "I know it sounds hokey, and I have never told anyone about that moment, no one." Why? I asked. He laughed self-consciously. "They would think I had gone off the deep end."

Many newly diagnosed patients do wander close to the deep end. Panic sets in. The path becomes blurry. Not so with Buzz. He took matters straight to the top. He was getting the situation wired with the Lord. By now in this conversation, Buzz had stopped chuckling. "Besides," he continued, referring to his pact with God, "it was private."

"What next?" I asked.

"I made sure everyone was okay, including the minister and the doctor."

"The doctor?" I asked in astonishment.

"Yeah. This was the radiologist who had to break the bad news, and he was not supposed to be the one to tell us. Our doctor had not done that." So, patient tended to doctor. "He said, 'Stop, Buzz. Let it sink in. Let yourself be angry.' I could not be angry. I simply told Susan, 'God and I have talked.'" Case closed.

BUZZ'S MEDICAL ODYSSEY picked up speed immediately after his diagnosis. The day after getting the bad news, he was at the Indiana University Medical Center in Indianapolis, meeting with an oncologist he would come to respect. Though Buzz's assorted earlier physicians had dropped the ball, this oncologist picked it up with sure hands.

"Boy, she was marvelous, smart, kind, caring, and very beautiful, by the way," Buzz said, adding, "and that was the fastest I have ever gotten my clothes off in my life, and she did not even ask me to." The doctor offered comfort and hope to the Bays. She built a relationship with the family that endures, though she has moved west.

The doctor immediately extracted bone marrow from Buzz's hip. "That was the most painful procedure in my life," Buzz recalled. "I bent the bed rail, it hurt so badly." Susan had been encouraged to hold Buzz's hand, because of the pain. "'No thanks,'" Buzz said Susan remarked, "'He will break it.'"

The procedure was vitally important. "This was to see if the cancer already had invaded the marrow," Buzz explained. "It had not. That is a good thing." And then? "Nothing." Buzz went through a slow-motion period known as watchful waiting. Doctors stand back and wait, monitoring the tumor until something happens.

It was a game of human chess. "The doctors wait for your body to make a move. Then they move. This was the worst time." In the Bay household, imaginations ran wild. "It sucked, because whenever you felt anything, you wondered if it was the tumor growing. If I got a cold or anything, it was, is this the cancer?"

The nerve-wracking period lasted six months. In April 2002, a CT scan revealed that the cancer had become active. The tumor was growing, invading Buzz's lower abdomen, between his spine and small intestine. "It had grown to the size of a baseball," Buzz said. The docs put him on the drug Rituxan. "The tumor shrank down to a little bigger than a golf ball."

The drug did not do much to alleviate the pain. Buzz explained that his tumor was free forming, meaning it was unattached and could move almost anywhere. "The pain is sporadic, but the mass can be extremely painful when the

tumor shifts and hits my spine. I just learn to live with it."
Too frequently, that is the story of chronic illness. Pain becomes a small price to pay for survival.

"I do have pain medication," Buzz explained. "I do not
like to take it because of the side effects, feeling woozy, you
know, not very sharp." He takes acupuncture treatments
when the pain is intense. "Usually, I just grin and bear it,"
he said with a broad smile.

"In May of 2003, I got horribly sick on Mother's Day,"
Buzz recounted. Now the guy had shingles. Shingles is
herpes zoster, a painful rash that produces an intense
burning sensation in the skin. Shingles is frequently triggered by chemotherapy as well as stress, and the pain can
be debilitating. In the summer of 2003, a scan indicated
renewed growth of the tumor, which meant more chemo.
"This was bad," Buzz said. "Shingles came and went, and
my hair fell out. I was sick, really sick."

Buzz is as decent a man as I have ever met. He practices
his beliefs through the six days that follow Sunday. He is
immersed in the word of the Bible. More than occasionally,
I have thought of the Book of Job. This book of the Old
Testament asks why, if there is a God, the innocent should
suffer when at the same time the wicked escape and are
permitted comfort and prosperity.

"Buzz, are you familiar with the Book of Job?" I
asked.

"My goodness, yes." He laughed. "At church, they call
me the modern-day Job."

"Do you believe you are being tested?"

"Yes, I do. Very much so," he answered quickly. "This
is all about how you deal with it." He paused. "God never

gives you more than you can deal with. Faith is always tested." Those tests continued, hitting Buzz from odd angles.

After my visit, we did not speak again for a few weeks. Then an e-mail from him popped onto my computer telling me that he had just been released from the hospital.He had gotten violently ill in the restroom at church. Susan had taken him home. "Then I got so sick, Susan rushed me to the hospital. I kept passing out. The doctor felt I could have had a mild stroke. I do not even remember Monday or Tuesday. My doctor came in and said she had not seen anyone so sick in her career."

When I called Buzz later, he told me his blood counts had suddenly bottomed out for no reason. He had been knocked out for a week, but finally was released and walked out of the hospital. It was a mystery. "I bounced back. It all comes down to the *F* word. 'Faith.' I prayed my way through."

The tumor was growing, and a week after the hospital stay, Buzz began radiation therapy. This wounded man would endure a total of twenty-eight rounds of punishing radiation, beginning before Thanksgiving. "I did not know what to expect," he told me during a subsequent visit as we drove around in his old van. This was high-tech torture. He lay in a sculpted form to prevent him from moving. A piercing buzzer sounded if he shifted even slightly.

"They put blue marks on my torso as a map." And? I asked. "I got burned, like a bad sunburn." The radiation did help. "It shrank the tumor some, but not as much as the doctor wanted." Buzz reacted violently. Treatments were relentless, concentrated in the lower belly, where nausea forms. "Gosh, I was very sick. They were cooking me." The vomiting would not end.

Buzz learned practical precautions to minimize the violent reactions. "Yeah, the hard way," he said. "You learn to eat very lightly. Usually, I ate about five meals a day. And I would sit down and just rest, just sit in a chair and not move. That was good." Cumulative pain and puking from chemo and radiation pushed him to a mind-set he had so far resisted: He felt like a victim.

"I had no options left. Seeing yourself as a victim does not feel right." The man's life was so miserable that he did consider, albeit briefly, halting treatment altogether. "The thought rested in the back of my mind," he admitted. "My goodness," he added, "this is not quality living."

"All along, doctors keep telling me the disease is incurable," Buzz said, "so why are we doing this, I mean, what is the point? I asked if he had resolved his urge to quit. "Not really. The thought never leaves the back of my mind." Buzz said his doctors had made clear that they would respect whatever he decided.

Buzz came to know the common emotion of many cancer patients. "I can see why people commit suicide. Pain and despair are so strong," he said long after his treatment ordeals. "Not me. I knew that in the end, faith would get me through this and make me stronger."

But God did not end the cancer or the pain. "No, but I found strength, and for me, that is proof that God is alive." As an article of faith, Buzz had to keep going. "We have an obligation to live that is moral and religious. We must keep fighting."

I have been prescribed drug therapies for MS that bring

on far less pain and discomfort than Buzz's. There are side effects, however, and I believe those drugs did little good. There was the strong temptation to quit. So I did quit, but only after years of telling myself, You never know. "That is it," Buzz exclaimed. "Maybe in some tiny way I will be better, and it will be worth it," he concluded. Then he added: "Maybe it will make the end easier. Just keep me comfortable and let me live the rest of my life."

I had not been thinking in terms of death, but Buzz's eye seemed focused on a spot that lies beyond his painful horizon. "Richard, heaven is going to be great."

"Buzz, I am not convinced we are headed in the same direction," I responded. "It may be warmer where I am going."

Buzz chuckled back. "You never know, Richard. You still have time."

However reluctantly, Buzz committed to continuing treatment. But he took a break. Thanksgiving and Christmas were fast approaching, and he did not want to be bothered with torturous treatments for a while. "I wanted to at least feel human again, to have some feeling of life and purpose. I did not want to put Susan and Ryan through so much confusion, you know, trapped on this roller-coaster ride."

Despite Buzz's wishes or wishful thinking, Susan and Ryan indeed are strapped in and along for the wild ride. With any serious chronic illness, families are sucked into the maelstrom. Meredith has often said in frustration, "This is not Richard's MS, it is our MS." There is no way to shield loved ones from the pain.

* * *

ON A FRIGID March morning a few years later I drove to Ryan's school near the interstate. A dusting of snow added shivers to the short ride to the outskirts of town. I had told Buzz I would be happy to talk to Ryan's classmates, many of whom were publishing little books in their third-grade classroom. The youngsters sprawled on small chairs, wide-eyed and focused. This was a guy from the big time, they had been told, and I was having a good time pretending that was so.

Even as various young students leaned forward in their temporary roles of aspiring writers and asked what it is like to write a real book, Ryan sat back, appearing disengaged. Kids shared their book ideas, some showing me what they had produced. Topics were age-appropriate, light-fare tracts about grandparents or sports. Buzz already had filled me in about Ryan's book.

"One day, Ryan came home from school and said he had something to show us. I thought he had gotten an F," Buzz remembered. Instead, Ryan presented them with a small, brightly colored, carefully illustrated book. The slim volume had been simply bound and self-published in his school.

Daddy's Adventure was Ryan's carefully crafted Book of Daddy and Cancer. The Bays had taken to referring to Buzz's anxious trips to the emergency room as his "adventures," hopefully easy listening for Ryan's uncertain ear. The concept stuck. The idea for the book had come from the boy himself, with encouragement from his teachers, but without the knowledge of his parents.

"I wanted to write about something I was feeling,"

Ryan had explained to his parents. "There are other kids with sick parents. Maybe this will help them." The book offered Ryan's take on Dad's disease. "Daddy and Mommy said going to the hospital is like an adventure," the book read. "When we see the oncologist, try a new drug, or have to stay in the hospital, it's like an adventure, something new and different to experience."

Daddy's Adventure is a child's attempt to demystify cancer. "Yes," Buzz said decisively, "it opened a whole new comfort zone for Ryan, that cancer was okay, that it did not necessarily kill you." Buzz was speaking with ease, as if in his own head he had worked this through. "You can live with the word 'cancer' or die by it, and together we have chosen to live."

Buzz and Susan had decided to speak openly with Ryan about Buzz's dealings with the disease. Meredith and I traveled the same road with our children, in the belief that full disclosure would foster security for them. I assumed Buzz had explained his belief that God is there for him and wondered if Ryan would stray far from his father's calming faith.

Faith in the face of illness continues to be a mystery to me. The belief that beyond the limits of medicine, God will take care of the rest involves an alchemical assumption spun from denial and faith. That confidence and the sense of peace it inspires reside deep inside the Bays as a family.

Buzz and Susan thought hard about what they were going to tell him about the cancer. "Ryan sat outside with us, quiet and attentive. That was very rare." Buzz laughed.

"I explained, with Susan on the other side, that I have a tumor and the tumor is cancerous. Ryan never cried. He asked if I was going to die."

"What did you say?"

"If it is my time to go to heaven, I will go and, I will be that angel on his shoulder to protect him. That seemed to work for him."

Buzz and Susan wanted Ryan to be prepared, not scared. Instinctively, the couple understood there is no alternative to the truth. "We explained everything," Buzz said, "and he knows where parts of the body are." They even told Ryan about the trouble spots.

"He knows what my blood levels are, and what that means. Ryan understands what a red blood cell is, what white blood cells are. He knows all that." Susan added, "We talk about the treatments and that sort of thing, and of course he sees Buzz sick. Ryan does see it, and he gets it, and that is good."

Ryan had been down this road before. Buzz's best friend, Mark, had been diagnosed with stomach cancer only the spring before Buzz's diagnosis. "That really bothered Ryan," Buzz explained. Mark was Uncle Mark to Ryan, who visited the trucker at home and in the hospital, laughing and crying with him as he deteriorated and died.

Ryan sees Mark in his father's suffering. "Oh, yes," Buzz said. "Ryan will see me sick and ask, 'Daddy, do you think you will go like Uncle Mark?'" Buzz remembered Mark's death as beautiful, but hard on Ryan. "Ryan sat in Mark's lap the day before he died. 'I will be watching you from heaven,' Mark told him. Ryan still brings that up."

Buzz believes that Ryan's calm adjustment to his cancer

did not connect to reality until the boy came face-to-face with cancer's brutal side effects. "The cancer did not register until he saw me throw up over and over after chemo and radiation. I was violently sick." Reality was reinforced when Ryan discovered Buzz collapsed in the church bathroom one day.

"He was so calm when he went for help that some folks did not believe him," Buzz recalled. "Ryan is very mature now. It makes me sad. He has had to grow up so fast. Cancer has been a part of his life for the last four years."

What we see on the outside, I have decided with my own kids, is not what you get deep within. Ryan's ordeal had to be more searing than Buzz could know or, perhaps, handle. Seeing his father's collapse in the church bathroom had to frighten Ryan.

"Susan and I talked to him and explained that Dad will get sick sometimes, but that the medicine helps him get better." Buzz believes that getting his son involved made a difference. "Ryan would read to me as I lay by the toilet with a pillow and blanket. He would be comforting me."

Buzz recounted one particularly bad bout that seemed to push Ryan over the edge. "Ryan flew out of the bathroom crying, 'Daddy is dying,' and he did it very loudly," Buzz said. "Ryan really was scared."

School counselors assured the Bays that Ryan was dealing with the family crisis well. Ryan's even keel could be temporary or just the boy playing to the audience around him, I suggested. "Handling the cancer well has stayed with him," Buzz answered. I was not convinced.

During my final foray into Indiana, I wanted to sit

down with Ryan to talk about the cancer in his family. Visits to the old farmhouse up till then had been casual and pleasant. Susan and Buzz knew of my interest in talking to Ryan. They agreed without hesitation. Not yet, I would tell them.

I had established, I hoped, a reasonable comfort level with the youngster. I wanted to wait for a moment when the boy was at ease, the conversation not forced. Ryan went along for the ride as Buzz and Susan picked me up at the airport for that visit. We pulled into the Bays' driveway and into the old garage. As soon as the car stopped, the boy was gone.

Buzz sat on the worn couch with me, patiently waiting. Eventually, Ryan came downstairs and sat on the floor at his dad's feet. A GameBoy was clutched in his hand. Ryan and I made small talk for a while, and then I tentatively began.

"Ryan, do you remember when you found out your dad was sick?"

"Uh-huh."

"Can you tell me what you remember?"

"Well, them telling me about it."

"What was that like?"

"I don't know." Ryan stared down at the GameBoy.

Already, the conversation was difficult. "Was it pretty scary?"

"Yes."

I looked down toward the floor. Ryan looked as if he was going to jump out of his skin.

The love in the Bay family is obvious. But Ryan seemed freaked, and Buzz needed to believe that the boy was just fine, that the cancer was not eating away at at him, too. I dropped the subject.

* * *

IT WAS 3:00 A.M. on an April day in 2005 when Buzz awoke, barely able to breathe, turning blue and struggling. "This was the first time Susan was truly scared," he recalled. "As we were going to the hospital I remember hearing Ryan say over and over again, 'Breathe Daddy, just breathe.' Susan called ahead to warn the hospital ER of what was happening so they would be ready." Buzz was relating the events in a totally unemotional tone.

We had driven by the local hospital numerous times during my visits to Franklin. The building sits just off a busy commercial street in the middle of town. It was not difficult to imagine that night.

"I was pulled from the van and Susan said my clothes were coming off as I was rushed to the trauma room." Was the place deserted? "Yes, but a great Christian doctor was on that night and never left my side. My stats were horrible, and at one point he did come to Susan with tears in his eyes and told her that there was nothing else he could do, and would she want me to go on a ventilator? Susan said that was the worst night, knowing that I might die. And there was Ryan. How would she tell him?"

Buzz and I were in the car, running errands, as the story unfolded. I asked him to pull into the hospital parking lot. People were wandering into and out of the hospital with no sense of urgency. "Did you think this was the end?"

"I felt like I was seeing everything from above and everything was in slow-motion. It was so strange."

"So what happened?"

"I cannot explain this, but like magic, my stats got better and my blood pressure came back up." I could guess the rest. "God must not have thought my time was then. I awoke the next morning in the ICU, wondering, How did I get here?"

"What were you thinking?" I asked.

"I just thought about how amazing God is. How can I use this for His glory? I was not afraid to die at that moment."

During the summer, Buzz suffered a partial bowel blockage, a by-product of the radiation. Doctors recommended surgery. Buzz vetoed the proposal because he did not want to be cut, thinking the cancer might spread. Instead, he opted for dependable discomfort until the situation rectified itself.

The doctors raised the possibility of a relatively new procedure, a peripheral stem cell transplant, with cells extracted from the blood instead of directly from the bone marrow. The procedure was less than five years old. The transplant was arduous. Even risky. Patients had to meet a baseline of strength and endurance.

Doctors knew that Buzz was weak and feared he might not survive the procedure. In the end, the decision would be his. He complained later to me about the manner in which the doctors presented options. "This makes me wonder, do the doctors ever talk amongst themselves or do the patients always have to intervene to get everyone on the same page?"

Buzz seemed to object to being offered more than one option. "Yes. Why can't they agree and just tell me what to do, what the treatment should be?" More proactive patients want options laid out, with an assessment of the upsides and downsides. These patients demand to be part of the process. Buzz wanted to follow orders, not weigh recommendations.

Finally, he was told in no uncertain terms by his trusted oncologist that a stem cell transplant would not be an option. "The doctor said I would not survive it," Buzz said, sounding peculiarly matter-of-fact about the whole thing.

"And that was it?" I asked. "No second opinions or further research?"

"No."

Some of us in the land of chronic illness object to rigid doctors who say it is their way or the highway and who insist on quiet compliance. Other patients resent having to weigh in on decisions that seem beyond their medical expertise. They show no interest in making decisions and prefer to follow orders by the experts.

Buzz does both. "Some oncologists get you, and it's like, it's their plan or no plan. They will not waver. This is what you are doing, and, no, you cannot do that."

Buzz claimed he had been aggressive, sampling unorthodox treatments and had to duck when he told the docs.

"I have met a couple of doctors who were like, well, why did you even try that?" It was the condescension that offended Buzz the most. "One just said, 'That is just a stupid old folks' tale, and who are you to say this?'"

Buzz defended his decision to experiment. "Too many of my friends have had cancer, and some have died. I cannot forget them," he said. "What the heck. This is my life and my body." He said a trusted doctor gave him advice he stored in the front of his mind: "Do not ever stop trying. Do what you think is right."

But Buzz is doctored out. He has decided to accept whatever fate awaits him. "Why be a guinea pig and put myself through all that and miss family time?"

Why not see another doctor and look into options? I asked one more time.

"No," Buzz answered with nothing in his voice. "I am okay."

This is cancer, man, I thought to myself. Do not be so passive. Learn more. Doubt. That was unlikely to happen, and to my mind, that was too bad.

Weighing options and participating in treatment decisions is what it takes to become a smart patient, a partner in care. Non-Hodgkin's lymphoma is a cancer with a menu of therapies. Assorted benefits and risks come with the selections made. I would not leave it all to the doctors.

I kept trying. We were driving through Franklin on a cold November day. I asked again if he could imagine traveling for an additional opinion. "No," he responded quickly. "Things are fine here." Passivity allows doctors, sometimes unnamed, to make unilateral life decisions.

THE DESPERATE EFFORT to stay financially afloat in a rising tide of medical expenses is the hidden story of chronic illness. The bills for high-tech therapy and costly medical procedures just keep coming, growing exponentially. At the same time, incomes can drop precipitously as jobs move into the background, taking a backseat to surviving another day after debilitating treatments.

According to a Harvard Medical School study, in 2001,

nearly 1.5 million American families filed for bankruptcy, about half of them citing medical costs. Even middle-class, insured families can fall into financial ruin, as sickness explodes and benefits run out.

By the close of 2004, Buzz's struggle had opened a new front, the battle of the bank. His medical costs were spiraling out of control. And his ill health was limiting his ability to earn anything that could be considered enough. Before long he was seriously in debt.

The new wound cut deep. A traditional man, Buzz found his position as master of the house, guardian of his family, diminished, and his spirit suffered. For him, a long-held passion pointed to a possible solution. Flowers. For decades, he had toiled in the wholesale flower business, working for others but always longing to own his own flower shop. He wanted to become his own boss.

When her husband became sick and sicker, Susan said to him, "Let's do it," Buzz remembers fondly. She recognized an opportunity for him to fulfill his fantasy. The Bays had to get beyond the *what if?* doubts. Susan wanted Buzz to have his moment.

"We bought the building and the business combined. It was a package deal with the bank," Susan explained. She and Buzz put up the equity in their home and took out a small business loan. They were in.

Buzz's flower shop was located in Greenwood, Indiana, just north of his home in Franklin. The shop was housed in a large yellow and brown Victorian on a quiet street. "The business got off the ground and flew very well," Buzz remembered with a smile. The Bays wistfully called the store Forever Flowers.

This small corner of Middle America was awash in colors and smells that belied the florist's beleaguered state. The bright scented flowers dotting the premises brought Buzz hope. "My spirits were up whenever I opened the door," he said. Flowers made him happy because they were for everybody and every occasion. Buzz told me, "I used flowers to marry people and bury them."

"You sound content when you talk about the flower business," I said.

"Those were great years," he replied, now characteristically fading into the past tense with a soft sigh.

Eventually the shop had to go. "The cancer got worse and basically took over," Buzz said. "I could no longer be nearly as hands-on as I wanted. I could not last for a whole day." Buzz also said that after the 9/11 attacks, the bottom dropped out. Along with everything else, the flower market went soft.

Buzz's business failure also had to do with loss of control. With good employees, perhaps he could have kept the business going through a dry spell. He paused. "Yes. Maybe," he answered, but "I could not get everything in the business done exactly the way I would do it myself. I am a horrible perfectionist," he admitted with a low chuckle.

Just as Denise needed to maintain control when none was in sight and her health continued to crumble, so Buzz couldn't bear to leave his business in the hands of others, even loyal employees. The Bays sold the business.

A man who teetered at the edge of losing his life lost a livelihood, too. "I felt like a total failure as a husband and father and, of course, provider. It was the worst time of my life," he said. "I was not able to say, 'Cancer, be gone.' I kept it inward, and I felt defeated."

Buzz cares deeply for flowers, but their colors and fresh fragrance are conspicuously absent in his warm and comfortable home.

"Strange, no flowers for you," I said.

"They are a luxury," Buzz replied. "It is like, eat or have flowers."

For him, the tough times got tougher. "I cannot get a full-time job at this point," he said. "An employer is not going to want an employee who is always running out for tests or treatments. It is unfair to them, but the whole thing is not fair to us." Frustration festers in him. "This situation was not our idea."

Buzz is not bitter that he has long-haul cancer. He is angry about the price tag. "We had planned for our twentieth anniversary to go to Hawaii," he said. "We were saving, but that is all gone because of the cancer. All our savings are gone."

Months earlier, a desperate fear for the future had poured into an e-mail to me. "Man, I have no idea where to turn. I have to come up with thousands of dollars and I just do not know where it is going to come from. No one wants an employee who might not be able to work. I have been told that a lot. Honestly, I am afraid for my family."

Buzz had made no attempt to mask his fear of homelessness. "What if we lose the house? What if I get worse? How are Susan and Ryan going to cope? Where are we going to have to live?" Buzz was learning to fear financial ruin more than the ravages of cancer.

"I am really scared about all of these things. Sorry to dump this on you, but this just keeps building. I lay awake at night just hoping for that miracle, that I would wake up and this was all a horrible nightmare. Susan can only work so much. Thanks for listening."

Buzz and Susan sought legal advice. "We are working with an attorney to do the bankruptcy thing so we do not lose our home," Buzz told me in a later phone call. "It is really bad. We owe over five hundred thousand dollars, and that is after our insurance." A number like that takes a toll on the head. "It plays with your conscience first," he said. "You know it is not your fault, but I was raised to pay bills and to never live above my means. It is mind-blowing when it happens."

Just leaning on a support system and asking for help challenge traditional notions of oneself as a man, but in sickness, independence and that male stubborn streak must be relinquished. They do not always go gracefully, though Buzz was grateful to others who could pick up the slack.

Susan's parents provided a reassuring though limited safety net for the Bays. The ride out to their ranch house on the outskirts of Franklin was pure Midwest, farms and tractors, terrain that stays utterly flat. The wind whipped across the prairie. No hills or buildings were there to stop the mean gusts.

Bob and Dorothy had become a vital two-person rescue squad for the Bays. "Oh, yeah," Susan exclaimed. "They pick up Ryan for us when I'm working and Buzz is working and stuff like that, and then after work I just go pick him up there. So that helps tremendously."

Bob and Dorothy's assistance is at once heartening and

distressing. Buzz knows he can turn to them if the bottom falls further. "They would be there for us. I know they would." The retired couple had greeted us warmly. Dorothy served coffee and cookies. "We are happy to do what we can," Dorothy said simply.

Buzz appeared uncomfortable. I could hear him gathering his thoughts as we sat at a traffic light on our way back into town. Farm equipment rattled through the intersection, and Buzz had to raise his voice. "I would rather we work things out for ourselves."

"Going to your in-laws for help would be tough for you, I imagine."

"It is hard," he answered. "Very difficult. It is like you are not supporting their daughter as she is accustomed to."

"No one has complained, Buzz."

"No, but they had put their trust in me. I feel I let them down."

Buzz feels compromised as a man, as a father. "If Ryan needs something for baseball, I just cannot do it. That puts a lump in my throat. You are not taking care of your family. That is how I was raised," he declared adamantly. "Take care of your family, and take care of their needs, and work. Period." He looked down the street. "I just try to stay alive."

"Buzz, you are nuts," I said. "I mean, you have cancer."

He laughed. "They all would say, 'You are crazy. This is not your fault.'" The nightmare of unrelenting chronic illness is that pride must yield to survival, no matter how you were raised or what you think is expected of you.

Buzz wears self-conscious vulnerability as a shroud, the burial garment of a man going under. Word of the financial struggle got out in his small community, and the melo-drama that followed makes for a good cry.

When the Franklin *Daily Journal* carried an article about the Bay family battle against non-Hodgkin's lymphoma, Buzz's struggle to survive was reduced to a cliché, a medical sob story. He learned how newspapers portray illness and the public reacts to soap opera on the printed page.

Buzz is not accustomed to wearing a public face. The article reported that he doubted that Susan would manage to make ends meet after his death. "He can't help worrying how his family will survive financially," the article read, "worrying that Susan's job as a secretary at the . . . hospital will not cover the home payments or medical bills."

"It was a freaking nightmare," Buzz exclaimed. He was humiliated by the publicity and offended, he said, by what he considered overstatements. "I am not going anywhere," he exclaimed. "The article sounded like I was checking out tomorrow."

He was particularly upset because the reporter focused on the fact that he and Susan already had planned his funeral. "There are certain things I want done, and without planning together, Susan would not know they should be done." It was as simple as that, he said, and not as morbid as the reporter had made it sound.

The Franklin community reacted with force to the story. "I got forty or fifty phone calls about why we have not been honest about my health and why we closed the business." Franklin is a village where people apparently either look out for one another or into their windows.

Buzz was reacting to a widening public view of intensely private circumstances in a community that already was manufacturing its own take on the story. The back fence was the local communications medium of choice. True or false, the story had legs.

The Christian community came together to raise money for the Bays. The event was a long time coming because up until then Buzz had very politely turned away helping hands. He was self-conscious about admitting to his precarious situation. Though Buzz was slipping financially, he seemed oblivious to the wisdom of Proverbs, that pride goeth before a fall.

Reality finally set in. "The bills just kept coming," he said. "Our minister, Larry, sat me down and had a heart-to-heart talk about how many people I have helped and that by not letting them do a benefit, I was robbing people of their joy of giving back to me and my family."

Buzz swallowed hard and agreed. "It was a strange feeling that night," he recalled. "People came with tears in their eyes. I felt like it was my wake. All the nice things people said, things that I did not think they even remembered. They were thanking me for changing their lives."

Buzz was caught off-guard. "I was taken aback by the number of people who came out that night. I never felt so loved. Realizing the number of lives I've touched was shocking, to say the least." And there was a lesson. "Sometimes the smallest of kindnesses goes a long way. God showed me that night that love goes deeper and farther than anything else of this earth." Maybe we are not as alone as we feel.

The benefit did help. A lot. Harder times would come.

* * *

CASUAL STOICISM HAD been Buzz's close friend. A strategy of not succumbing to high emotion allowed him in his own mind to move forward. He wanted to stay on a higher plain, to remain above the fray. This stance made him seem disengaged from his cancer. It was unclear how aggressively he intended to fight.

Buzz's brand of passivity either reflected a deep inner peace or belied sheer terror. His silent struggle was known only to him. He claimed to feel no anger, not at the cancer, not with God or his fate. He was even quick to forgive the reporter who created the embarrassing article about his collapsing condition. "I was just disappointed. I do not get angry. I know she wrote from the heart. It was just one of those things."

There was no anger for the doctor who dallied with the diagnosis and forced his patient to go it alone. "You know, to this day I have never been angry at anyone," Buzz says. "What is there to get angry about?" I could think of a lot of reasons, but they would fall on deaf ears.

"I think attitude is ninety-eight percent of the battle," Buzz often said. "Keeping positive is so important. Maybe you can take control of your body with a positive attitude." He would have no problem finding smart, secular people who believe in the mind-body connection.

Buzz's insistence on locking his emotions away worries the people in his life. Susan is frustrated by his reluctance to reveal himself, perhaps even to know his own emotions.

"Ryan and I can tell when something is wrong," Susan told me, "and we want to know what is going on." It sounded like the taciturn culture that I knew in my family, growing up with a sick and silent father. My old man has MS and actually invented stoicism. At least, that is what I've come to believe.

Whatever brews in Buzz's brain, no cry of "poor me" will pass his lips. He demands that the world see him as what he wants to be, not what cancer has made of him.

"Buzz needs to take care of other people," Susan observed. "That is part of his makeup." Selflessness comes to him at the expense of emotional health. "I do not think he takes care of himself emotionally here on earth. His goal is to go to heaven. I know that," Susan went on. "And he is going to go his own way."

Buzz's solitary silence irritates Susan. "It makes me really mad," she said forcefully. "Sometimes, I would just like him to say something when he feels bad, you know." She turned, as if facing her husband. "Why don't you just say, 'This is a bad day for me. I feel sick'? It is weird keeping something like that from me."

This had been put to Buzz before. "Buzz gets angry when I tell him." I pointed out to Susan that Buzz told me he never gets angry. She smiled. Sort of. "Well, he does not really show it. He just gets upset when we call him on it," she said. "Ryan and I know when to back off."

I asked her if she could understand how chronic illnesses can stretch couples to the point of splitting them apart. "Sure. The spouse gets tired of the stress day in and day out. If they are not open, a lot of people cannot take it."

"And you?" I asked.

"I am not sure how we get by."

It came back to their traditional faith. "We took wedding vows, you know, for better or worse." The commitment between Susan and Buzz survives unquestioned. A life has been threatened, but the marriage is meant to live on. "Buzz and I take our promises to God seriously."

Disease and divorce can travel together, and the toll is undeniable. All among us hear the horror stories.

My firefight with colon cancer seven years ago burned Meredith and singed the kids, but the fight had a beginning, middle, and end. Chronic illnesses such as Buzz's have long if not endless middles. The conclusion of my struggle was happier than Buzz's promises to be. We survived on our own brand of hope. Susan and Buzz have plenty of fuel on the fire to keep that flame alive.

TO HELP OTHERS die in peace has become a calling for Buzz. More than ten years ago, hospice workers had tended to his mother as she lay dying of breast cancer. He started working as a hospice volunteer in 2005, and a year later, hospice officials invited him to join the staff as the paid volunteer coordinator. He works three days a week. Hours are flexible, to suit his physical needs. "I work at my own pace. They are very protective. If you do not feel well, you do not have to worry."

Paid work brought the sun back. "Oh, my." Buzz sighed. "The job gave me self-worth. I was a man again." That he found work became a banner headline in his mind. He become a professional cancer coper, and reclaimed his self-respect. He was back in the game.

Buzz was gleeful that at last he could take part of the financial load off Susan's shoulders. "This is huge for Susan," he said with pleasure. The position, though no guarantee of winning enough bread for every meal, was a shot in the arm for both of them. He began to feel more hopeful. Choosing his words carefully, he said, "For a cancer victim, hope is like winning the lottery."

"Well, you know the odds on that one."

"Yes," he laughed, "but see, I can hope, too." We sat at the dining room table, silent for a moment. I could hear Susan telling Ryan something up the stairs. "Hope is that the next day a cure can be found," Buzz continued. "Maybe the next day, a gene will be recognized by some research scientist, who says, 'Let's attack this gene.' That is going to stop lymphoma. That is going to be the big answer."

For Buzz, hope said it all. "Hope is the ballgame of life," he observed, "because if you lose your hope, if you lose that, then you just want to give up. Without hope, there is nothing." Hope in a hospice has to be hard, but Buzz seemed to find much satisfaction in his work there. "My wife says I want to know what it is like," Buzz said, "how people react at the end."

He joined Susan in acknowledging that probably he did need to watch others die to prepare himself for his journey away from this life. "I cross the bridge with them. I have held their hands as they pass. If I have helped to make someone's life better, I have done my job."

"What do you get from this?" I asked.

"I feel a sense of peace."

More power to him. The hospice did seem an appropriate place for Buzz to accomplish his personal mission: to remove fear from dying. It was almost as if he had been guided to the spot. He would tell me he was.

* * *

DURING MY FIRST visit to Franklin, Buzz and Susan and I piled into their van and embarked on a tour of the quiet streets. It was a weekday morning. There were no people anywhere. "My Lord, the churches are everywhere," Buzz exclaimed. "Just look down the street," he said approvingly. "There is Baptist, there's Presbyterian, there is Pentecostal, there is Mormon, there's Methodist." And we had not turned a corner. "We are in the Bible Belt," Susan added.

The sheer number of sanctuaries amazed me. "God is everywhere," I said.

"Of course, my friend. Down here, there is not just one, but all kinds of Baptist, Southern Baptist, and Northern Baptist."

"They are all separate churches?" I asked.

"They are all separate churches," Buzz verified. "A lot of churches that are nondenominational are livelier than ours, more charismatic."

"What does that mean?" I asked.

Buzz explained that these churches really rock. "They just let go," he said, "with shouting and wild singing. There is hand raising and clapping." He stopped for a moment. "I like variety," he added. "We go to all these churches sometimes."

"What do you get from that?" I wondered out loud.

"There is a kind of an awareness of other Christians, a renewal." Buzz plays a set role in his own more conservative church. "At these other churches, I can worship the way I want, be myself," he said. "There is good fellowship there. Our church is great but not at that point."

At those sanctuaries where there is live music, perhaps

Buzz does let go. "Stuff does build up and, wow. Oh, it offers a huge release," he said with enthusiasm. "Susan does not care for the charismatic movement. That is okay. I sometimes go to one of these churches alone or sometimes with Ryan. There is a cleansing. It is like my therapy."

"It seems as if one or another of God's varied drumbeats keeps you going," I observed to Buzz.

"It really is faith," he responded.

I stared at him. "Faith in what?"

"God," he said immediately.

"You believe God will help you?" I asked.

"I am certain," Buzz answered without hesitation. "I will be cured in this life or in heaven." I know. That assurance had become Buzz's mantra.

Later that day, as the Bays and I bounced along in their van, a CD on the seat next to me caught my eye. I reached for it as we pulled up at a traffic light. The album was called *Amazed, a Journey of Faith*. There was a photo of three guys in front of a brick wall looking their Bruce Springsteen best, informal and intense. There, in the middle, stood Buzz. He had said nothing about the CD, just leaving it for me to discover.

"So you are the yodeling florist," I said.

"You should hear his voice," Susan said. "It is great."

The recording is well done. "It is a journey of faith, my friend. / Step by step, He's with you, / His loving knows no end," went the title song. "He'll chase away your darkest days and fill them with amazing grace. / Leave behind your yesterdays and today start a journey of faith."

The CD was recorded in 2002, well after the cancer diagnosis. "The whole group knew the possibilities," Buzz explained, "but we decided to keep singing our music 'til we can go no longer." He said the CD was an independent project that paid for itself.

"Did the recording have anything to do with your illness?" I asked.

"Only that I wanted to have something to leave Susan and Ryan," Buzz answered. "Something with my voice on it." Each song in its own way became a statement of faith.

It struck me as odd to hear relatively young guys sing about God with such conviction. My cultural association with faith goes to old folks heading around the bend. Buzz wrote one more song for the most important member of a new generation, a fair-haired boy who pads around his own house.

"Oh, how he prayed to you, as he prayed for me. / He knew without a doubt, you would answer my needs. / So Lord I come to you. / I don't know what I must go through, / but I will trust in you like I see Ryan do." Buzz's song for his son made clear that his faith has been passed down.

Christianity reaches deep into the Franklin community and is the defining piece of the culture for residents of all ages. This is the bosom of the Bible Belt. The citizens of Franklin are God-fearing, Jesus-loving Christians. For Buzz, Christianity is not part of life. It is life.

"You have to have faith to live around here," said Kim, who with her husband, Craig, owns the Ashley-Drake, the local bed-and-breakfast where I stayed during each visit. Buzz had wanted me to stay there. The young couple displays no religious symbols on the walls of the quaint old place, no outward signs of their faith, but that faith was evident as we sat over coffee at an antique oak table. Christianity was their frame of reference, and it crept into many conversations.

The Franklin Memorial Christian Church is a large modern structure that looks as if it belongs in a shopping mall. The church serves as tabernacle and part-time theater. The sanctuary is immense, housing religious services and hosting Christian cultural events. The church is almost a complete world for its congregants. Buzz goes to one, sometimes two services on Sundays. Church events and activities fill out much of his remaining week.

Buzz's devotion to his faith and church together is the linchpin of his life. A true sense of community is pivotal to him. No one wants to go it alone, and here he has found a spiritual sedative that gets him through the night. And though a nonbeliever such as I finds this focus on faith rather hard to accept, the church community is seductive. Communal caring can grow on anyone.

On one clear, cold night in December, I attended church with the Bays. It was shortly before the Christmas holidays, and Buzz had to jockey for a parking space. The pageant was the biggest show in town. I had set off to visit the Bays because Buzz wanted me to see Ryan play a Wise Man and hear him sing a solo in the Christmas spectacle.

The evening had the feel of a rock concert, the Stones go to church, with laughter and small talk and refreshments for everyone. These were people who were important to one another, individuals who touched each other's lives.

These were Buzz's people. I watched the man work the crowd, hardly a politician seeking votes, but an ordinary guy drawing sustenance from others. "You okay, Buzz?" punctuated the evening. A hearty handshake or silent squeeze supplanted the need for more words. Buzz smiled that smile and drew it all in. The scene played out in stark contrast to Denise's chosen isolation. This church had become one man's therapy. Buzz moved with ease, his complete faith and easy deflection mixing seamlessly, faith and denial coexisting comfortably.

Buzz's minister, Rev. Larry McAdams, Larry to all, sees through the cheerful dance Buzz carefully choreographs for his audiences. "Buzz needs to talk about himself. He needs to tell someone how he feels. He reaches out to others in need. That is great, but . . ." But what? I wondered. Larry's frustration with Buzz reads as tough love. "We ask Buzz how he is, and he comes out with trite little things like 'They haven't got me yet' and 'I'm upright and taking nourishment.' I say, 'Buzz, that is not good enough for me.'"

The reverend said Buzz avoids him sometimes, backing away from conversations he does not want to hold and, perhaps, emotions he does not want to face. "With illness or tragedy, anger is appropriate," Reverend McAdams pointed out. Larry reminded me that Jesus said, "Be angry and sin not," meaning, be angry, as angry as you want, but hurt no one with your rage.

Buzz, according to his minister, needs to face the music. "I do not think he levels with me or anyone else about what the doctors are saying. I do not know if Buzz has accepted the fact that nothing is going to save him."

The reverend suggests that Buzz might be bargaining with the Lord. "Maybe Buzz really thinks God will prolong his life if he helps others." He paused. "I have never seen anything like Buzz in thirty-six years of ministry,"

Larry concluded. That was a powerful informed assessment.

Larry McAdams has been at this kind of work for a long time. Where the good reverend and I perhaps lose our footing is that I figure if Buzz is going to die soon enough, let the man do it his way. There is nothing that suggests to me that there is any benefit in facing the cold, hard truth, according to the terms of others. What is the virtue of staring yourself down in the mirror and emoting for its own sake? If we allow others to tell us how to live, they will want to tell us how to die. Their truths would not set Buzz free. Coping becomes whatever works, even if, for Buzz, that means joking too much and falling back on faith.

I respect those who find the faith that eludes me, but envy is not part of the package. The Almighty never cut me any slack, issued a rent check, or bought a sweater for me when I was shivering. When I was hungry, I fed myself. And here was Buzz, dropping every egg he could find into the bottomless basket of faith. His life was moving not so slowly in a bad direction. Yet the man believed that somehow the Lord would intercede and all would be made whole.

Even when his brother suddenly died, Buzz toed the line. "My brother is at peace," he told me calmly. "He is with Mom and Dad and my sister up in heaven having a great old time." He chuckled. I was long past the point when anything Buzz said surprised me.

This man's faith is so complete, heaven so alluring, that death seems but a bend in the road. "Heaven is an incredible place where a lot of things and people, humanity, our family and friends are." My friends ask all the time if I am envious of Buzz's strong faith. I envy the peace faith gives to Buzz, but I cannot get there.

"Please tell me about heaven."

"It is a place that is beyond anything I know, any pictures I could paint. There is no camera shot I could take that is more beautiful or more outstanding. There are no words that any poet could ever print." I was mesmerized by the description. "For me, death is the gateway to a life of no pain, no worries. I will get to see people I miss, hug and live with them forever. How can that be so bad?"

"You really do believe that, don't you?"

"I always have believed it. I have no fear of death." There is a different fear. "I have a fear of leaving my family, but I know their faith will sustain them." Buzz broke the spell with a laugh. "I think Susan will say, 'Give me two weeks and I will be back out on the road, looking for somebody else.'" Buzz thought this was funny. "No," Susan interrupted. "Yes," Buzz answered. "First time, go for the love, and then go for the bucks."

"Nice to see you laugh, Buzz. I just would be angry."

"I know you want me to say that I am angry. I am not. This is just a brief stay on earth, and we all die. Through this trauma, I will shine for God and not look back. God knows our needs before we do. We cannot fool Him. I have not led a perfect life, but I have been forgiven."

A STARBUCKS SITS conspicuously along Route 31 going into Franklin, standing alone among the gas stations and greasy eateries. My pumpkin latte and the eighteen-wheeler parked outside seemed a visual contradiction in terms.

"Buzz," I asked, "has the certainty of your faith made you accepting of death and led you to stop fighting?"

"That is a tough one," he said, pausing. "Since I know where I am going, I am not discouraged to die."

"Really?"

"Yes. I know you will think I am crazy, but I am excited to go."

"I already think you are crazy, Buzz," I replied. "Then why fight it?"

"Because of Ryan and Susan," he answered. "That is it." Then he threw in one additional thought. "The only selfish motive is this. I do not want to be forgotten."

Perhaps Buzz was not as immersed in denial as those around him are wont to believe. He did at times show flashes of anger, faint lightning in the distance. "I am angry at the disease for robbing me of so much stuff," he finally conceded. "Obviously, yeah, I do get angry with things. I get, like, Why is this happening now? What purpose does it have? Why did I get this way?"

Our conversation was animated and loud. I looked around Starbucks and realized some folks were staring at us. Buzz told me that my presence in town had been duly noted.

"Buzz," I kept on, dropping my voice, "I get mad for the same reasons you claim you should not. The angry response has little to do with logic or even faith. You can believe in God and still feel that you got screwed," I continued. "You did get screwed. So did a lot of us. Maybe I am only attempting to justify my own life in a bubbling cauldron. Boiling over from time to time does present one big release. Get pissed off just once. Don't laugh it off."

"Humor to me is part of the way I exert my negative energy," Buzz said. "My anger is in humor. When I get nervous before I go in to the hospital, I start laughing at stupid things or making stupid jokes. Laughing makes things that are so horrible to people like us okay. We laugh and know God is there with us."

For Buzz, God slips into every scene of his drama. He would rather talk about God than himself. "I am guarded," he admitted with a self-conscious laugh.

"Why are you guarded?"

"I do not want people to see my vulnerable side," he explained. "I am not the strong person I want other people to think I am."

"Doesn't your hospice work show you people's vulnerability close up?" I asked.

"Yeah, I am a witness to emotions that I will have when I go."

"Doesn't that make it easier to let down your guard?"

"I want people to say, 'Buzz is strong.'"

"Then it is an act?"

"Yes," he blurted out, though with the utmost calm. "You can take it as an act." Buzz needs to be seen as the strong, silent type, though he is hardly at a loss for words. "I want to be the rock," he said, "to take care of others."

"Buzz," I ventured, "we all want that. Perhaps now it's your turn to be cared for."

"I don't want all this poor victim stuff," he replied quickly.

"Who said anything about poor victim?"

"I hurt," Buzz told me suddenly, as if, finally, I had cracked through, or maybe just worn him down. Keep going. "Sometimes the pain from the tumor is overwhelming. The hurt just takes over. But who wants to hear about that? I listen to folks complain about aches and pains, and they have no idea," he exclaimed, referring again to his own searing pain from the tumor.

"Look," he assured me as he hit the emotional brakes and skidded to a stop. "I am at peace."

"Buzz, that is beginning to sound like a cop-out," I said.

"Not really. I think I know my limitations, not that I want to be prudent," he said back to me.

"Meaning?"

"Meaning, I stop at a certain point and do not go further."

"Why?" I asked.

"People will care to a point and do not want to hear everything." Buzz was right about that. "This complaining stuff is out of my element. Do you understand, Richard? It is very hard to give up control. This is a control issue."

Bingo.

The loss of control becomes the common complaint of the sick. Take a number and get in line. There are a lot of us fighting that battle. Look at Denise. After my thirty-something-year crusade against two debilitating chronic illnesses, I have never made my peace with ceding control. That gradual hemorrhaging goes on. Buzz can control his emotions but not the disease. You take what you can get.

BUZZ CALLED ON a weekend. There was more bad news. Job was back in town. "The cancer has gone to my cerebellum," he said, with no trace of emotion. The cerebellum sits in the back of the head between the cerebrum and the brain stem. It is responsible for movement and balance.

"How did you find out?"

"I had an intensive MRI. The cancer has become more active. We knew this could happen."

"What next?"

Buzz chuckled. "We will take each day and see."

I thought I could hear the shrug of his shoulders through the phone. "I am fine." And Susan? "Susan was weepy. She had been away. I picked her up at the airport, and she knew something was up," Buzz said.

Susan would not get into the van until he told her what was happening. She was so upset she needed to run back into a restroom to cry alone. "We went to our Bible study later that night. Twelve close friends were waiting there." These were a core group, friends who know everything about one another.

"Did that provide comfort?" I asked.

"Very much so," Buzz answered. "These are very strong Christian people."

Buzz underwent a spinal tap.

"When do you get the results?" I asked. "In a few days," he said on a Friday, meaning over an endless weekend. A tense time? "I am at peace." Right. It was clear that he was expecting bad news. He quietly believed the cancer was spreading. For now, all he could do was wait for the phone to ring.

And ring it did. For two days, as I tried repeatedly to reach Buzz and Susan. They were nowhere to be found, their house seemingly abandoned, their cell phones turned off. On Monday, my call to the emergency room where

Susan worked yielded an unembellished "She is not here." A reintroduction and explanation for the call prompted the nurse to pass along a private phone number upstairs in the hospital.

"Buzz had been sent home after the spinal tap, and later in the day he told me he was not feeling well," Susan explained in a weary voice. "Suddenly he passed out. He could not talk." She said she was so flustered she could not seem to dial 911 and asked a friend to make the call for help. Buzz was unconscious for more than an hour. Susan thought he was dead. So did Ryan. The child had screamed hysterically, "Daddy's dead! Daddy's dead!"

This was only another weekend for the Bays. The family had grown used to these unexplained events. Susan put Buzz on the phone. "Hey, guy" was about all he seemed to find the energy to say.

"Are you wrung out, Buzz?" I asked.

"Yeah."

We agreed we would talk again in a few hours, when he had seen the doctor and had a better sense of what was going on.

I reached Susan later at home. Buzz was in surgery, undergoing another spinal tap. This time blood from his leg would be injected into the tap site, creating a blood patch to prevent the leakage of spinal fluid that had caused him to lose consciousness days ago. He would not be going anywhere today.

"I do not know why it is me," he said the next day. "It is very odd. Things are progressing. We will know more soon when we get the cytology report." He said the only therapy left for him is a procedure called sudden-burst chemo, which may slow down the cancer. "This is not a cure," Buzz pointed out. "It can help with the pain. That is what we are left with."

Again, watchfully waiting, Buzz stood ready for his story to play out. Long ago, he realized his journey was about to change. He saw a better place and knew deep within that he would be there. His only question was when.

BUZZ WAITED FOR the next event in his body, and he dreamed. Those dreams, visions, he called them, came in recent years and, he said, brought warmth and peace into his life. He had said little about them to Susan, almost nothing to anyone else. The first vision came to him in 2002, after a rough round of chemo. He was in bed in the middle of the night when something happened.

"There were three entities. I cannot put a face on them, but all had male voices. Their appearance was brief, and I just thought it was the drugs." Was it? "No," Buzz quickly answered. "If it happened once, maybe it would be the drugs. This would happen again and again." There was a message. "They just said I will be going to a far better place than I have ever imagined in my life." He said the voices went on. "'But it is not now. It will be in God's time.'"

He wondered what that meant. "What was said to me was that all would be revealed in time."

"How did you react?"

"It scared me." He chuckled. "These were persons, but there were no faces. Over time, it has calmed me down."

Through the years, entities would appear, if only to assure Buzz that his time on earth was not done. The reward, he was assured, would be better than ever he could expect. "I kept thinking these are tricks of my mind, my imagination. I needed to tell someone."

Buzz told his minister some of the story but wanted me to talk to him about the rest. Larry was unflappable. "I have talked to different people who have had similar experiences over the years. These stories are not unheard of," Reverend McAdams told me. "So many things are unseen by the human eye. I believe there are angels and demons. The Bible tells us we are in a war with things we cannot see. God talks to us in different ways."

The visions were not just late-night events. One sighting occurred in broad daylight. "Once I was at home in the lounge chair," Buzz said, "and Ryan came in and said he heard me talking to someone. He thought someone had stopped by to see me." Buzz remembered Ryan walking around the corner and seeing no one. "I asked him, 'Ryan, where did the three men go?' Ryan told me there had been no one in or out of the house."

"And what did Ryan say after that?"

"He said, 'Dad has gone nuts.'"

Another vision came in 2004, during Buzz's painful kidney shutdown. "The men comforted me, saying I will get through this. They showed me a place that was so beautiful no one could imagine." What was it like? Buzz faltered, reaching for words that would not come. "It was the most, well, stunning and beautiful, glamorous place on earth. Triple that," he added.

He was hospitalized in early 2006 with the flu and a possible stroke. He was unconscious for two days. Another vision came. "I saw my Mom and Dad, family and even close friends that have gone on before. They assured me again that my time will be soon, but in God's time. They told me they will bring me home."

When he passed out from the pain of the spinal tap, once again he thought he might be setting out on that journey home, getting ready to see his family and friends again. "Our choirmaster was my friend Dan, who died of hepatitis C. He and my friend Mark were there. They looked so real and so beautiful. Their bodies were just incredible, not like I remember when they were so tortured and racked with pain. It was awesome to see."

I called Reverend McAdams again, reaching him on his cell phone in what sounded like a crowded, noisy place. "Is it possible," I asked, "that Buzz has created an image of heaven drawn from his culture, music and movies and magazines, and invented his own final resting place, complete with three wise men?"

"Yes, it is possible," Larry answered evenly. "And is it possible the Lord was speaking to Buzz and comforting him in what may be his final hours on earth?" he countered. "We do not know." Larry was displaying his usual patience with my doubts. "We will never know."

"Is it important," I continued, "to know which is true?" I did not wait for Larry's answer. "No," I said loudly, so the good reverend could hear me in Indiana. Buzz was finding his peace. That really was all that mattered.

Most of Buzz's visions appeared in times of crisis. They became his port in the storm. Visions arrived as he lay unconscious or when he sat alone in a hospital or at home. He did not know if the end was fast approaching. Perhaps this man was writing parables for himself, his script for departing on his own terms.

These were his untold stories. For him, heaven would be lush and green, forever alive and in exploding Technicolor. Heaven would be breathtaking. "Heaven," Buzz said, "will make Oz look like the Bronx." He laughed his laugh.

"I know people will think I am crazy, or that it was just the drugs or my imagination," he said, "but I know it happened, and I know in my heart that God truly loves Buzz Bay. God has his angels with me all of the time, and that is why I am not afraid to die. Richard, I hope someday you can experience what I did. It will change you forever."

Reflections

Honoring a Separate Peace

Perhaps the most powerful lesson of my many trips to Indiana was the danger of having a closed mind. Too often we become captives of our prejudices and narrow in our outlook. Buzz, the man under my microscope, was taking me at face value. My mistake was not to afford him the same courtesy.

As a smug, godless New Yorker, I ventured into the Bible Belt expecting another human being to deal with a life-threatening illness on my terms. We all think we have the magic down pat. I had learned to cope with illness my way, doubting authority and leaning on my hyper-rational and dispassionate self. What I was ignoring was that this formula worked for me, not for Buzz.

We cannot dismiss the faith of another, though that seems to be in vogue in the world these days. And there I was on the town square, condescending toward the man from whom I should have been learning. My mind did creak open, and I let go of the judgments that had no rightful place in this inquiry.

Not all of us are serious Christians. But I learned to admire Buzz for having a set of principles and living by them, even if his wrinkle-free thinking was hard to accept. If the sick flounder, perhaps it is because we get too caught up in our dramas, unaware that in fact we have anchors that keep us grounded in the storm—and they are uniquely personal. When we recognize our own anchors, we can accept that others' differ but might be equally effective.

Buzz's time on this planet is spent in service to God. He is selfless in his everyday dealings with his close Christian community and is prepared to leave his family in their care when he hits the road for sunnier climes. That Buzz is ready, if not eager, to set off for heaven makes him glow. What greater peace is there?

four

Ben Cumbo

Facing Down Demons

THE SNOWFLAKES WERE fat and wet, falling halfheartedly through a gray sky over Kent Hall as a ragtag army of students moved through the old building. On this blustery late March day, the Cultures of Africa seminar was supposed to begin mid-afternoon.

At the appointed hour, young men and women straggled in, but there was no professor and no sign of Ben Cumbo, my subject on this day. The place reminded me of all the college halls that had incarcerated me in my years as a reluctant student. Undergraduates were fidgeting in worn seats as if they would rather be anywhere else.

Getting to Saint Mary's College of Maryland had not been easy. The school is a remote outpost, resting above the St. Mary's River at the southern tip of the state. Buildings sit close to the point where the river's brackish water joins the Patuxent and flows into Chesapeake Bay.

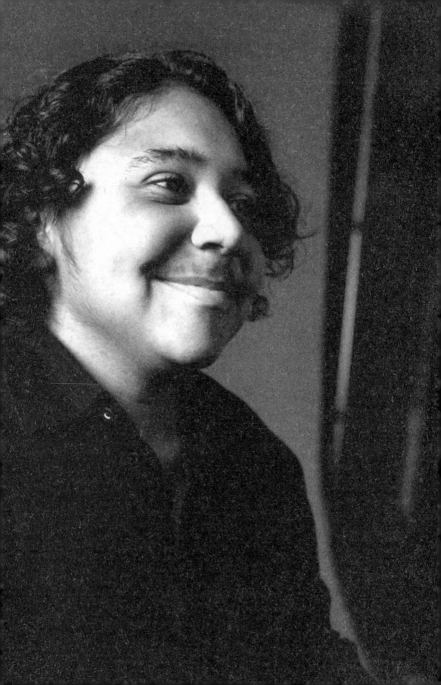

"You can't get there from here," the saying goes, and had been offered as a warning by my friends in Washington, D.C. They were not kidding. The college is not accessible by public transportation from the nation's capital or anywhere else. Only an old buddy traveling in the same direction got me there.

We drove south from Washington on highways leading to smaller roads winding through the countryside. These country roads deposited us in surprisingly rural terrain so close to the big city. The school was surrounded by farms and fences, with the giant Patuxent naval station looming in the distance.

I walked around Kent Hall, lurked in the hallway outside the classroom, and scanned the young faces, searching for Ben. Finally, as Ben's teacher approached the classroom, a mass of papers in hand, I heard an elevator door open and turned. The signature hum of a motorized chair was audible, announcing Ben's arrival. Ben looked up, silently nodding.

Ben was a good-looking fellow, with strong features and intense dark eyes. At eighteen, he was small for his age, though that was not immediately obvious because he spent most of his time in a wheelchair that was both his prison and his liberator. Ben's size was the side effect of regular steroids that might prolong his life but had stunted his growth.

Ben's wheelchair was a mean machine. "Can that thing go fast?" I had asked at a previous meeting. "It moves." Ben had chuckled softly. "Out in the open, on a smooth surface, you would not be able keep up with it." No kidding, I had thought, glancing down at my cane.

Ben performed a quick 180° in order to leave the lift and head to class. In one smooth motion, he shook my hand as he rolled by, gliding past the others milling around the large seminar table. He had mastered precision, executing tight turns and swinging around to position himself near the professor. The maneuvers seemed effortless. I slipped into an empty seat next to him, sitting in silence for a moment as we waited for the seminar to be gaveled to order.

To say that Ben was quiet or understated is its own understatement. The guy was borderline silent. I had learned over the past year, through visits with his family, that conversation did not come casually to him. There was a pronounced self-consciousness that I had to work through whenever we met. It was almost as if his shyness were another chronic condition to overcome.

"When Ben gets going on a subject, he can go on at length," his dad had told me. "When it comes to talking about himself or his life, he does not have a lot to say." Ben's father is Benjamin Cumbo III, Big Ben to me. I so wanted his son's discomfort to end, though thus far it had not.

"I have never been to this part of Maryland," I said to young Ben in a forced whisper. "This campus is pretty cool," I added, leaning in toward him. "Yup," he responded, eyes straight ahead, not even glancing at me. "It sure is in the middle of nowhere," I offered up. Ben just smiled. Okay, then. Maybe the stilted conversation was due to our age difference.

Ben was but eighteen then and I, let us just say, three times that. Ben is African American, and I, Caucasian. We had not found our comfort zone, and personal conversations were awkward for both of us. Ben was in the starter's gate, a disabled kid facing his first adventure away from the security of home. Time together made it plain that he is quietly angry, but so am I. There was a lot to talk about.

In this particular seminar, the discussion deconstructed various African subcultures, their customs and rituals. The content as well as the mixed demographics of the classroom—black and white, rural and urban, privileged and not—introduced Ben to a level of diversity that he was only slowly getting used to. How are we different? was the professor's question.

Sitting close to Ben, I took note of his seriousness and the level of his concentration. During this two-hour class, more than occasionally, he took risks, asking and sometimes answering complicated questions no one else was touching.

When papers were returned to the students, Ben sat back apprehensively, waiting to see how he had done. His writing project had focused on the Shluh, a North African people and culture centered in the mountains of Morocco. Ben grabbed the paper from his professor, painstakingly reviewing the comments on each page. His face revealed nothing. I waited for him to say something, but his concentration went unbroken.

Finally, I leaned toward him once more and asked how he had fared. "I got an A minus," he answered, finally betraying a small smile. There was no sense of celebration in his voice, no expression of satisfaction. "Well, an A minus is great," I said. Again, there was silence.

"I do not want to lose my edge," he explained later on the phone. "I want to do a better job next time. I am pretty much moving on to the next challenge." The young man radiated discipline. But why so serious? I asked.

"I agree that many kids my age would have reacted more," he said. "I have this work ethic. I force myself to buckle down. When I complete the class, the whole thing, then I will celebrate." I found that hard to believe.

"How did you choose that topic?" I inquired in a whisper.

"I was interested in indigenous belief systems before the domination of Islam." Huh? This kid is more disciplined and serious than I was at that age.

Ben only wanted to continue his discourse on religion. He was a Methodist by birth, but, he said, "I do not consider myself a Christian or Jew or Moslem. I just know I believe in God and take the good things where I see them." He went on. "I am learning about my roots. It is interesting, cool to see where your ancestry starts, you know, where you are from."

Ben is a true and earnest student who clearly loves being in college. His interest in Africa was intense. This second-semester freshman was 100 percent there, entirely focused, even as other underclassmen were showing difficulty recovering from spring break.

To Ben, the brief break had meant little more than an opportunity to catch his breath. Others in the class spoke about sleepless drives to Florida, of beaches and parties. Ben had spent the week at home, readying himself for his return. I was convinced that young Ben was compensating for the frailty of a damaged body by exercising the muscles of his mind.

For him, education and preparing for an uncertain

future seemed a grim business. Completing his uphill battle, proving to himself and his doctors that he could move into adulthood, was the challenge at hand. Any youthful enthusiasm was missing in action.

BEN SUFFERS FROM Duchenne muscular dystrophy. The diagnosis came when he was just three years old, too young to understand. His parents were not. Big Ben, a swarthy man with a graying beard and hair, was a defense analyst who had spent thirty years in the Pentagon. Ben's mom, Debi, stayed home briefly after her son was born, returning to her marketing job at *USA Today* until her daughter, Tyler, came along. Debi is straightforward and easy. She describes herself as stern when necessary, a pushover when there is nothing at stake. Debi now works for the American Council on Education.

Tyler Cumbo, three years younger than Ben, is a freshman at Hampton University in Virginia, a predominantly African American school. Big Ben's daughter from a former marriage, Erin, is eight years older than Ben. Erin attended Howard University in Washington, preparing for a career in architecture.

Young Ben's ancestors, he would learn with interest, probably came from the western coast of Africa. Ben himself hails from Upper Marlboro, a town in Maryland just outside the nation's capital. Ben grew up in a quiet middle-class neighborhood. The Cumbos' community used to be predominantly Caucasian. But white flight had worked its magic, Big Ben noted, making it more African American.

The Cumbo family's journey into the land of illness began on Super Bowl Sunday in 1991. "Ben was a chubby little guy, very much a toddler," said Big Ben. "He was in a preschool with another boy whose father was a doctor at Children's Hospital in Washington. They invited us to watch the game at their house."

Details of the chain of events remain clear. "The day after the game, I got a phone call from the doctor. We talked for a minute about the game, and then he made an observation." Big Ben paused. "He said, 'There may be nothing to this, but I noticed how Ben was going up the stairs.'"

Big Ben responded with little concern. "'My son does seem to move around a little differently,'" he recalled saying. "'Yeah, he will not be a major league athlete or anything, but we are taking it as developmental.'" Big Ben said the talk was low-key. "The doctor said, 'Maybe, but why don't you set up a couple of dates at Children's for him to get some tests?'"

Big Ben was not worried about his son. "Ben was slower than the others. He did lag behind other kids when they were running. It was not a big thing. I just figured he is not going to be a speed demon. There was no indication. I mean . . ." he looked away as he trailed off. "This was a perfect little boy. He was laughing, running, the whole nine yards, and he took care of his infant sister."

Recognition of an illness can come slowly, awareness beginning with subtle signals. The Cumbo story called up memories of a day long ago when I dropped a coffee pot and fell off a curb. Those minor incidents led to a clear-cut diagnosis of multiple sclerosis. The Cumbos thought there was no cause for alarm. "I was not worried," Big Ben reiterated. "I just was not."

The senior Ben recalled a series of tests on his son done

in one day, procedures that generally take one week. "To make a long story short, at the end of that day, the doctor called us in after reading the results. She told us, 'There is a seventy percent chance that your son has muscular dystrophy.'"

Big Ben said his blood ran cold. "Those two words linked in my mind to Jerry Lewis and the telethon. I was oblivious at that point as to what the disease was and what it meant."

"This was news from nowhere."

"Right," the older Ben affirmed. He spoke slowly, reconstructing his disorientation. "'What is this?' I thought. 'Where does it go?' I remember this woman doctor talking to my wife. I was in a total haze of confusion." And the numbers game began. "I was just . . . things were going through my head like only thirty percent chance he is okay? Tell me what that thirty percent is, what it means."

The doctors, Big Ben said, were straightforward. "At first, they were great." There would be more tests, first a muscle biopsy. Doctors said that would pinpoint what the problem was. Getting results might require as long as six weeks, which became its own horrifying prospect.

The boy's parents spent their time researching the disease. They were riding an emotional roller coaster. "It was total angst the whole time," Big Ben remembered. "There was a sense of panic, actually, wondering, how do we adjust if this is true?"

High anxiety travels with any looming, life-threatening illness. "'Angst-filled' does not get close to it really," he said. "You've got to get through your day. I was at the Pentagon itself then, and I was overwhelmed." Ben's emotional openness surprised me. The man had been hanging out with defense types, hardly known for their candor, for his entire career.

The six-week wait did not materialize. The call came within ten days. The Cumbos found themselves back in the doctor's office. "It is amazing how the visual plays in your mind."

"How so?"

"Professionally, I am in a visual world. Maps and photos and satellite images," he explained. "The intel [intelligence] business is all about bits and pieces being put together." I did not understand where this was going. "We walked into the doctor's office, and there were drawings in great depth. It was an omen."

"Of what?"

"The drawings are not there if the news is good." Big Ben's sixth sense was on target. "'We are certain that this is muscular dystrophy,' the doctor announced." I could sense Ben's emotion rising. "'We feel ninety-five percent certain.'" Everything in medicine seems to be hedged in percentages, sort of like handicapping a horse.

"'There are three kinds of muscular dystrophies,' she went on." Ben's exasperation shot over the top. "I said, 'What is the worst muscular dystrophy?'" Ben says the doctor was silent for a moment. "'This.'"

"This" was Duchenne muscular dystrophy, the most common form of the disease. It causes muscles in the body to become very weak. In little more than a decade, they can break down, replaced by fatty deposits. The illness leads to the inability to control vital muscles. There are few experimental treatments and there is no cure.

Duchenne usually is fatal in the teenage years. "Give me a break here," Ben recalled thinking. "Everything is coming down, man." His eyes welled up as he relived that moment. "The doctor quickly realized that my wife and I needed to be alone to deal with the whole thing. She left, and we emotionally just . . ." Ben paused. "We were confused. There were all these things that go into finding out something so devastating."

It was over, yet just getting started. "This doctor came back in, and then she started telling us things we did not want to hear." Like what? "She told us what would happen, like a wheelchair by age eleven, respirator by fifteen, succumbing by the age of eighteen. She wanted us to know the whole thing."

The Cumbos were appalled by their specialist's rush to painful predictions. In the next minutes, the couple backed away from the doctor with the dark crystal ball. "That doctor went to the Genghis Khan School of Medicine," was all Big Ben will say about her.

Among the chronically ill and their families, complaints about doctors know no end. Physician as soothsayer is one of many outrages. We can only wonder how deeply these doctors care or even know about keeping hope alive.

"I think that the doctor was wrong to say those things," I said to Big Ben.

"It is all related to bedside manner, if that is what it can be called. Luckily we had our friends at Children's Hospital," he replied. I wondered if he had expected better. "I did," he said. "Then."

The Cumbos moved on, finding a new, more empathic physician. "This doctor backed away from reducing the illness to inevitabilities. "He was optimistic. He said things like, 'Yes, that could happen, but the statistics are changing daily.'" The ability to mix realism with hope is a precious skill.

BEN AND DEBI understood there would be a rough road ahead for their son and the entire family. They were determined, however, to lead young Ben into as normal a life as would be possible. They wanted him to reach out instead of giving in to illness. The Cumbos were determined that their son have dreams.

"He wanted to be a railroad conductor," his dad remembered, "and then a pilot." Dreaming allowed the young man to see a future, to be able to imagine in the midst of high emotion and confusion over where he might be headed. "Ben's dreams allowed him to focus not just on what he could not do but on fantasies of what he might want to do. That was critical." What the boy would reach for became more realistic through the years.

Ignoring grim possibilities was easier to accomplish in Ben's early years, with the disease progressing slowly and Ben's recognition following at the same pace. "I wanted to be a fireman or policeman, things like that," said young Ben. "They were the normal things that every young boy would think about, say, between the ages of five and nine."

Learning the diagnosis and understanding the problem were gradual. "I want to say I was five when it registered."

"Were you surprised?"

"Not really. The information did not have much of an

effect. I knew that I was different, but I did not grasp how devastating it would be." By the time he began to feel the effects of the muscular dystrophy, Ben was old enough to understand. "Until then, I felt like an ordinary kid."

Instinct suggests that early disclosure usually is the right call. Ben's parents dispensed information about his illness gradually and in small doses, carefully assessing what their young son was ready to absorb. "There are levels of truth," his dad said. "What we told Ben at five was different from what we said at ten or fifteen. At five, it was, you have a disease that affects your muscles. That is all."

The boy's parents did not know from one day to another where the disease would take their son. "In the beginning we said that anything bad would not happen for a long time," Big Ben said. "It was kept vague and in the future."

"We told him it was a progressive disease," Debi remembered, "but the doctors said he was doing well."

The difficulty explaining an uncertain future to a child is obvious. Ambiguity can be unacceptable to a kid. As a young adult, I found it hard enough to get a handle on MS when no one could tell me where it was heading. The long-term prognosis was dark, but the Cumbos hoped for some light. "We just decided to take each day as it came," Debi explained. Young Ben's eyes opened slowly as the severity of the disease became apparent. As he reached second or third grade, his legs began to weaken. He was tiring easily, though he was still able to get around on his own. The sinister signs of his illness were kicking in.

Young Ben described emotions with characteristic understatement. "I did not react in a positive way," he said ruefully. "I was upset." As always, he offered a perspective that was surprising for his years. "It was not physically as difficult as it is now."

When Ben was still walking and independently mobile, he could sense only vaguely what lay ahead. "At times, I thought about the future, but not all the time." His even keel may have floated on the easy denial of a child. "I pushed away reality, like probably all children do. I chose not to deal with things that made me worry."

Although his parents were pushing for normalcy, they understood that integrating illness into his identity was the next step. Big Ben and Debi intended for young Ben to see his disease as a piece of himself and to make him as comfortable with his illness as possible.

Young Ben was introduced to advocacy work when he was eight, learning at an early age the value of getting involved and meeting other young people with the same problem. The Cumbo family became active in the local chapter of the Muscular Dystrophy Association, doing volunteer work and participating in the local telethon. The Cumbos' efforts to help other stricken kids drove home to Ben that he was not alone in this disease.

Ben was affable, impressing a Muscular Dystrophy Association representative. The boy became the Washington Goodwill Ambassador for MDA. "Ben understood what this was all about," his dad said. "He was helping people." At least that was the message Mom and Dad were trying to send. Then the Cumbos were approached by the national organization. The youngster was now under consideration to be national Goodwill Ambassador. MDA sent a camera crew to Maryland to videotape the Cumbos at home. The advocacy group dispatched the family to Boston to meet Jerry Lewis, the famous father of the mother of all telethons, where he was performing in a revival of *Damn Yankees!*

"Everything clicked," Big Ben remembered. Young Ben was singled out as a national ambassador. The family appeared in cities around America. The honor empowered Ben and became a first step in his taking charge of who he was. "At that point, it was a fun experience," said young Ben. "I was meeting people and going on television. Later, I knew it was more than that. I learned about going out of my way to help others and trying to change things."

A few years later, young Ben found himself on Capitol Hill, testifying before a crowded Senate appropriations subcommittee hearing on health, chaired by Sen. Arlen Specter of Pennsylvania. Ben was the small boy at the large table, dwarfed by the tall microphones.

He was comfortable in the spotlight. "I am just a regular thirteen-year-old boy," he told the senator, "just trying to get a girlfriend, listen to hip-hop. Do everything a thirteen-year-old boy would regularly do." Then the young man got serious. "I am extremely lucky, and God has blessed me because there are people who are a heck of a lot worse than I am."

Then the ball sailed over the fence. "If the government could spend two billion dollars on one plane," he said, referring to the B-1 Bomber, "a hundred million on research would not hurt." That line, no doubt supplied and rehearsed, brought down the house. Young Ben was learning to deal with an adult world.

Ben was not going to become a professional victim. His

parents were adamant about that. "I do not look down on people who make that choice," Big Ben said, "but I recognize there is a very thin line here that people deal with on a regular basis. We simply did not go there."

Young Ben was emerging with a strong sense of self that embraced his disease. "Keep your friends close," the Godfather warned, "your enemies closer." Muscular dystrophy was the enemy, but Ben was tacitly agreeing to live with it.

THE CUMBOS WERE careful not to make their other kids casualties, either. Young Ben's elevated public profile caused no conflict with his sisters. I sat with Tyler and asked if her brother had a corner on attention. "They would call Ben up and give him all this stuff," Tyler said, "but I never saw that as him being treated better than me." This pretty young woman was at ease. "Getting involved meant a lot to all of us."

Discipline was meted out impartially. When the siblings were young, all of them would get in trouble, including young Ben. Tyler laughed at the memory. "It was not like my dad would punish me but not him. Ben would get the same punishment, you know, no computer, no telephone. We were not treated differently."

There is a clear culture of success in the Cumbo family, and no one was exempt from great expectations. The kids were pushed to do their best. Tyler excelled in basketball, young Ben in writing. And they were supportive of each other. "Ben was at every single basketball game, just cheering," Tyler said. "I don't think it ever affected Ben in a way where he was like, 'Gosh, I wish I could do that.'"

Tyler wore a thoughtful look. "Ben was excelling in

writing all these different stories and all that stuff. I wish I could be a writer, just like him."

"Do you think it bothered Ben that you were so good at things he could not do physically?"

"I think it probably helped him a lot more because he saw me excelling in basketball." Her success pushed and inspired him.

"Absent Ben's illness, we would have had the same expectations," said Ben's father. "With the disease, that is even more the case." Why? "The alternative is not consistent with what we have always told any of them, to remove obstacles and make a difference."

If the Cumbos were intent on treating Ben as normal so he would regard himself the same way, neighborhood kids were not necessarily on the same wavelength. It is no secret that kids can be cruel to one another, often unintentionally.

"Remarks that other children would make drove home the point that I am not necessarily normal, at least the way they are," Ben admitted. "'Why can't you walk fast?' 'Why do you walk so funny?' or 'How come it takes you a long time to get up?'" Ben described the remarks as frequent and hurtful.

"Of course, those were the innocent observations of little kids."

"Probably," Ben answered. Still, he felt emotionally bruised. "People probably do that because they do not know, but I started to be like, okay, this really does hurt, and this is something that I want to go away."

Ben's parents could not help. "I would not necessarily say they prepared me. I kind of prepared myself. We talked several times about why certain people act a certain way, but it was ultimately up to me."

Ben said that at times his fears would subside, but the worst fears became his emotional Achilles' heel. As the boy became a young man, he became obsessed with the judgments of his peers. His fear of others became his demon, coinciding with the realization that his physical problems would amount to more than a bump in the road. "I learned that this thing was something that I would have to deal with longer than I had expected."

"What do you mean, longer?"

Silence echoed for a moment. "Longer means the rest of my life."

In a state of serious sickness, acceptance of a limited life can arrive in a slow drip, especially when we are young. At first we resist any knowledge of our limitations. Then, little by little, we let the truth in, particularly when the insensitivities of others are thrown at our feet. Says Ben, "I guess gradually I began to accept it and be, like, okay, I am not going to be able to do what I thought I was going to do as a little boy."

YOUNG BEN ATTENDED Bishop McNamara High, a parochial school with a predominantly black student body. The Cumbos are Methodists but thought the school would offer their son a better education than the local public school. I spent a long morning at Bishop McNamara during Ben's senior year, hovering around students and attending classes.

We ate a lovely institutional lunch that day, French

fries and more French fries. For me, this was a trip down Memory Lane, consuming what passes for a meal in a noisy school cafeteria. This time, I just watched. Ben seemed to let go of his customary serious demeanor, chatting away, even shouting along with the others. For the moment, he blended in, just another kid.

Akili and Glenn sat close to him, bookends supporting each flank. The two were his confidants and buddies, the guys who got Ben to come out of the house and lead a life apart from his family.

Virtually every face around the table in that lunchroom was black. The kids' easy camaraderie was obvious. Ben let down his guard to belong. In sitting position, legs under the table edge, he became just a member of the club. The festivities ended with the bell, and students returned to more serious pursuits.

Ben's ambitions had ratcheted up as high school was winding down. The young man was determined to be a writer. "A very successful writer," he said, clarifying the plan. And a famous one. "I want to be known by a lot of people as that screenwriter who is young, maybe twenty-five years old."

Success as a writer would provide affirmation that he was a whole person.

"Yes," the young man agreed. "It means that after bumping heads, I have cracked through. It means I am winning the war."

"Who are you at war against?"

"This war is not with other people, but the fight against the demons within myself." He went on. "I am fighting anger and self-doubt, spawned within myself and magnified by disability." Who writes this kid's lines? Above all, it was clear that Ben needed to believe in himself.

For years, Ben had been writing short stories, most of them built on military themes. He seemed to be taken with combat and strategies, men overcoming obstacles while operating under great pressure. His fiction seemed a metaphor for his life, an idealized snapshot of the kind of man he longed to be.

"If Ben were one hundred percent healthy, he would be in the military," Debi had told me. "That is his concept of being a man." What this mother cannot know is if her son is glorifying what he knows he can never be. "Exactly," Big Ben said. "Exactly. I say to him, son, you write in a context that is romantic and has a movie flavor to it, but that is not real life."

The real world may not be where young Ben chooses to hang out. "Escapism" is not necessarily a dirty word. What does Ben gain from embracing reality? Ben's parents were wary of his need to escape. I asked them what their son gets from reality. "Depression," they answered in unison. "If you look at it hard, you might ask, 'Why bother?'" Debi added. "'Why get up?' 'Why go to school?' 'Why do anything?'"

"Are there answers to those questions?"

"Yes. That kind of existence is unacceptable. You have to keep going."

Ben did keep going with his writing, expanding his themes and developing ideas that went beyond military heroes saving America. With high school graduation and college approaching, he worried about losing old friendships and facing the challenge of the future alone. For him, the subject inspired a work of fiction, *King Me*. Loosely based on his life, the book sounded his concerns as he prepared to leave the safe place he called home. *King Me* tells the story of close friends going out into the world, trying to do well by doing good.

The book has four principal male characters. Three bear the names of Ben's closest friends: Akili, Glenn, and Thomas. The fourth is fictional, based on the author's view of himself. The four band together in a group called The Disciples, who dedicate themselves to solving life's toughest social problems. The young men devote their labors to ethical dilemmas and sorting out religious conflicts. The heartaches associated with disability win their attention. The four vow fealty and go into the world, though they continue to meet annually, presumably a scenario of great comfort to the author.

Each of the disciples forms an organization. Akili's organization, The Core of Joy, is the linchpin of the group's shared social conscience and reflects Ben's personal concerns. The Core is a support group that takes up the large challenge of helping people who suffer from disabling diseases.

Disability is Ben's curse, yet in his book he made it Akili's cause. Would it have been difficult to make the story more autobiographical? "It would have been tough. Maybe taking it on myself would have been therapeutic." Ben sounds as if he was not interested in the role of single-minded advocate.

The fictional organization he created presents advocacy as Ben thinks it should be practiced in an ideal world. "I wanted to show that there are ways to make life better, even for the disabled. Yeah," he said slowly, "I have a duty to talk about this stuff, for myself and for others."

King Me, Ben's elaborate dream, works on paper. "I know I have created the polished look of what four young and successful African American guys want to be. Definitely," he said. Ben is well aware of the difference between fiction and nonfiction. "It may not be exact, but to be successful is the key to life."

As *King Me* makes clear, Ben's creativity and drive for success are unusual for someone his age. But the idea that his imagination has been hard at work is not surprising for someone whose body is failing. There undoubtedly is a correlation between loss of the purely physical and the ascent of the mind. Taking up residence in the mind is common among the disabled. There, we are free. We can explore and go places our bodies cannot carry us.

That transference is Ben's story. The mind picks up where the body leaves off. "Definitely," Ben said enthusiastically. His voice was animated. "I know what you mean. If one sense is taken away, others are heightened. That is beginning to happen to me."

Erin and I were talking about her younger brother over coffee in Washington. The bright-eyed young woman believes that Ben does compensate well. "I think that people who have physical disabilities have other gifts in other areas. I have seen that in Ben."

That observation marinated over time as siblings watched one another and matured together. "I am not physically blessed," Ben said. "When I look back at situations that were hard to overcome, I realize that in the end, I win out in different ways that take time to see."

Debi and Big Ben created their own publishing imprint to put out *King Me*. The book finally was published during Ben's freshman year at college. Afterward the couple decided to broaden their horizon to look at the work of other young African American writers.

At a reception for the new author at a local inn near the Cumbo home, friends and relatives were joined by college officials and even local politicians to honor Ben. The Cumbos were well known in the community for their advocacy work.

There was an *aw shucks* quality to young Ben's public face as guests sang his praises that afternoon. The contrast between craving a following and pushing away the attention was apparent. In his head he had needed affirmation from others for so long. When it came, he shrugged. "I guess it is not so important."

Ben's smile did not waver, though, the sole signal of satisfaction he allowed himself.

AT ST. MARY'S on a snowy day, I watched in wonder as Ben tripped the light fantastic in his motorized wheelchair. He rolled through Kent Hall, pushing buttons to open automatic doors and moving decisively, gliding backward and forward. Then he nonchalantly set out to cross the campus.

Ben had located the paths to avoid, scoping out the hazards, the holes and curbs he could not climb. He had identified shortcuts and knew precisely where to slide past parked cars and when to take the long way around. This was a survival game and he was intent on winning.

We started down a steep stretch toward the bottom of

the hill. As we approached the main road that cut across campus, I imagined what disaster could await. Ben could find himself slipping and sliding into fast-moving traffic. "You okay?" I asked. Ben shook his head and laughed, as if danger were his business.

Winter in a wheelchair is no laughing matter, a lesson Ben already had learned the hard way. Weeks earlier, he had been hungry, heading off alone for the campus store. "There was a lot of ice on the ground, and that made it treacherous." And the slow slide down a long hill began. "I thought, 'Oh, my God. What have I done now?'"

He remembered the helpless feeling as the chair lost traction and away he went. "What went through your head?" "Don't panic yet. Hope the chair just stops." It did. The lesson? "Do not go out in the snow," he answered sheepishly. Like I said, this is a game of survival.

Ben lives a life of anticipating trouble and plotting to avoid whatever disaster lurks. "You've got to be extra careful. In my head, I am the same as everyone else, but there is a lot more to think about with physical stuff."

Ben's parents thought about his physical needs early on. They bought a traditional ranch house with no steps just one year after the diagnosis. When a disability is present or foreseeable, planning is essential, and the Cumbos wasted no time. The house was easy for Ben to navigate. He grew up on his feet and remained standing until his mid-teens, exceeding the expectations of his doctors.

When he was in high school, his legs began to seriously weaken. At sixteen, they finally failed, decimated by the disease and the aftermath of a devastating auto accident.

Young Ben was a passenger in a car driven by his grandmother. A collision took her life and left her grandson unconscious. "It was tragic," Ben's dad said about the loss of his mother and his son's injuries. "We all believe that Ben deteriorated on his left side and was never the same."

His son agrees. "I guess that not using my body after the accident made the disease worse." The arrival of the chair came quickly after that. "Yeah. That accident did put me in the chair earlier. I believe that." The transition was tough. If young Ben appreciated inevitability, that made it no easier.

"Initially, I resisted," Ben admitted quietly. "There was a big old pride issue. I did not want to admit I needed help. But I could not walk anymore." And there was one more powerful incentive I totally understood. "I did not want to risk being even more embarrassed by falling all the time."

A comfortable, slightly worn chair replaced Ben's legs. A motorized chair moved him around, even as his peers were taking driving tests and moving to the driver's seats of automobiles. If a new car is a point of pride in our culture, the wheelchair is a signal of weakness in a society that celebrates physical perfection.

The irony is that though to the public at large the wheelchair is a symbol of dependence, for the disabled, the rolling seat, in fact, is the opposite, an instrument of freedom. Ben had lost his legs. The high-wire act had to do with reconciling his loss with the freedom he gained.

"It was tough. I am not going to lie. I was worried about what people would say," he said. He wondered how he would be treated. His nervousness was predictable. Long ago, a young man in a wheelchair had complained bitterly in a PBS documentary I helped produce that people only see the chair, not the man in it.

"Do you ever feel ignored as a person?" I asked Ben.

"If they have gotten to know me, hopefully they say, 'Okay, this guy is cool. He is not a chair, he is a person,'" Ben said, sounding surprisingly casual. "'He is not a part of some piece of machinery. He is an actual human being that has thoughts and dreams and goals and stuff that he has set for himself. So why bother disrespecting him?'"

Ben's fear was overstated but would not go away. "The effect was nowhere near as detrimental as I thought, because people automatically were, like, more sympathetic and stuff, like, 'Oh, he's serious with this. He has a physical problem.' I guess most people thought, 'Okay, we need to help this guy out,' and I think most people that I knew adapted to that."

The young man was learning to take his finger off the trigger. "I guess I changed people's attitudes toward me." Ben began to regard others with less suspicion. "I learned that nobody is out to get me." And? "I realized there is always someone around who has it worse." Amen to that, brother, a coping device straight out of my arsenal.

"There are deaf and blind people out there. I learned to count my blessings."

"You learned that pretty quickly," I pointed out.

"It was a crash course. I was forced to change, to ask for help. It was bound to happen."

Asking for help is not so easy, especially for those of the male persuasion. There is a tension between coveted independence and the willingness to reach out and say, Please.

* * *

BEN IS OUT in the world now and on his own. Life in a chair means that he has to rely on others. Only when he goes home does he know the security of a place he has mastered. One autumn afternoon, I walked through the family house trailing him.

The guy made his way in the chair from the bedroom, through a hall, past the living room, and into the kitchen. Obstacles were passed at close range and with ease, corners and doorways negotiated gracefully. For all the mobility and freedom a chair can offer, life without the use of lower limbs is fraught with difficulty.

Finding his way into the wheelchair each morning requires upper body strength and agility. Lying prone in his bed, Ben must stretch his arms up and out to reach a horizontal trapeze bar over his head. He pulls his torso and limbs to an upright position. "Since I cannot get up from a sitting position, I basically rely on that mechanism to help me up."

Ben must go up and out. "I swing from my bed to the wheelchair and get to the restroom or to the shower and back again." He sees the lift in calm, commonsense terms. "It is something that I very much need, because there is still some degree of independence for me. I am capable."

The system, though laborious, works easily enough when the chair is properly positioned next to the bed. One day, Ben's parents had left early for work, his sister Tyler for the gym. Each had neglected the regular check to establish that the chair, in fact, was in place for Ben's morning acrobatics. No chair, no chance. Ben awoke in an empty house to find the chair out of position.

He calmly stretched and reached up for the bar on the lift. With one arm grasping tightly to the bar, he slowly lowered himself to rest his knees on the floor. Then he swung toward the motorized chair. He was able to activate his machine and guide it toward the bed. He then used the lift to return to bed and begin his maneuvers again, this time the right way.

"You must have felt like a baby trapped in the crib."

"No," Ben answered immediately. His hard tone told me that my observation was off or at least uncomfortable. "I did not look at it like that. I had the lift positioned next to the bed and knew what to do. I was going to deal with it," he said, adding, "No big thing."

Ben will not admit weakness or vulnerability. He paused. "I am not suppressing anything. I was just taking care of business. My mind goes into the go mode. It just takes some ingenuity."

There are reprieves from the wheelchair. Ben goes vertical when getting into or out of cars. The young man is lifted, arms under his shoulders and hoisted by the strong backs of Mom or Dad or close friends. Observing the ritual of Ben being moved into and out of the family van took my breath away.

His legs were swinging and swaying, moving from side to side like a pendulum or just dangling like a rag doll. I worried that two generations of Cumbos were going to go flying, but the precarious look of the maneuver was deceiving.

The Cumbos are used to this high-wire act with no net. Ben rides shotgun, next to his mother. I realized the young man was seeing his world from the same high perch as anyone riding in a van, a welcome change for a guy in a chair.

I wondered if Ben ever forgets that he is sick. "Yes," he replied without hesitation. "There are times I do not think about the wheelchair. Sometimes, I am just one of the guys." Does that feeling of liberation last? "Not really," he said with no apparent emotion. "Enjoy the moment, I tell myself. It cannot be maintained."

BEN's COMFORT ZONE in his African American world vanished when he left his community for a predominantly white college. "It was a blessing and a burden," he said. "I am getting a picture of the real world now." There was a brief pause. "I feel intimidated."

He claims the experience is forcing him to shed labels and open his mind. "After a while, I become just a student." You mean, as opposed to a black student? "That's right. People help each other and gain from it. Maybe it does not matter so much."

I wondered how this young student sees himself. "Ben, you are male, black, disabled. As you define yourself, in what order do you place them?"

He paused and answered firmly. "I would have to put disability first." He started to say black was next but corrected himself. "Male would be second," he said instead, "then, African American." African Americans are about 20 percent of the student body at St. Mary's. "Yes, and that is disappointing. But there are only two students with muscular dystrophy."

Ben might have veered to his racial identity. He was a proud young black man. That he chose disability as first was a small surprise.

"What do you think Ben's order was?" I asked Big Ben.

"African American first," he answered without hesitation.

I met Ben's sister Erin at a coffee shop in the Adams Morgan neighborhood in Washington and asked the same question. "He said African American. I am sure Ben said that first." Erin laughed, smelling a trap.

"No," I told her. "That is what your Dad guessed."

"Really?"

"Yup. So did Tyler, who thought that being black would trump the others."

That the family missed Ben's reasoning points up why we, the disabled, can feel so alone. "Disability is the most standout feature of my life," Ben had said firmly. Disability dominates the mirror. The physical problems become what we see. Our imperfections take over who we come to believe we are. Limitations loom large. Even our loving families do not get that. They see what they choose or need to take in and process.

The Cumbos have been processing sickness at close range for close to two decades. The senior Cumbos are role models for families dealing with chronic illness. They have learned to go with the flow and adapt to all contingencies on a daily basis. That attitude has served them well as a coping mechanism.

"I feel that I do not get by," Big Ben had told me when

his son was in high school. "I get through. My job is to find a way to get through a day." A pause followed as the man collected himself. "Getting through is for him and the others." Big Ben said he had routines and rituals to try to make his peace with young Ben's disease.

With his son at home, his father would wander down the hall to Ben's bedroom. "I go to him. He may be in his room, at his computer. Sometimes I just lie down in his bed." Ben described a quiet connection to his namesake.

"What do you get from being with him like that?" I asked.

"I find solace. Somehow. We are together." I wondered if that intensified the terror of a young life threatened by disease. "My deepest fear is him preceding me in death." He is haunted by that very real possibility. "These moments with him ground me. I am more together. And I feel less anxiety about, 'Is this going to be the day?'"

Big Ben manages to get past that question. "On a couple of levels, faith controls all in our lives," he said. "We learned to pray and reach out. We felt we had to maintain a true relationship to God. 'Please do not put our son through this,' we prayed. We wanted the doctors to be wrong."

In a video prepared a decade ago by the Muscular Dystrophy Association, Debi described the crushing blow to the family that came at her son's diagnosis. "The thought of somebody telling you that you are going to lose your son when he is just getting into adulthood and you see just all of your dreams and hopes taken away from you . . ." she trailed off as the camera kept running.

Her husband picked up the narrative on the video, offering an emotional description of what his family had endured in those early hard times. "It required a lot of searching in our souls, a lot of restructuring in our lives," he said simply. "It was difficult, but we made it through that period."

With tears in his eyes, a younger Big Ben went on to explain how the family had survived the crisis. "We made it through the strength of our faith, our belief in God. We gave that task to God. And he has taken it for us."

I told Big Ben about Buzz in Indiana and how strong his faith is. "Buzz's relationship with God is his life," I said, "and he is very open about that." I pointed out to Ben that I had not heard him mention faith the same way. Ever.

"I consider faith to be very personal. I keep it to myself because I do not know how others will hear it from me." Perhaps he was sensing my different attitude about the role of religion in recovery. Unlike Buzz, Big Ben seems to see faith as a piece of his life, not life itself.

Young Ben had told me he believes in God but eschews organized religion. But is faith an important piece of coping? "When you are sick, you do feel like you are by yourself." The young man seemed to be searching for an answer here. "Religion does not have a lot to do with it," he said.

"I pray, but sometimes I just leave it alone." I said to Ben that it sounded like praying was just to cover his bases. "I can pray all I want, but I do not believe it will translate to anything." Again, there was that pause. "It goes back and forth for me."

"When I was sick, especially with cancer, and at my

wit's end, I would scoff at religion. What has God ever done for me? I would demand in anger."

"Yeah," young Ben agreed. "Sometimes I get mad at God, but then I don't think I should. At that point, I rely on faith and think about how bad others have it."

Young Ben seems to be walking both sides of the street here, full of doubt but playing it safe. Unlike his father who lives by hope and seems to believe that doctors will find answers in time to spare his son's life, young Ben's agenda seems secular and pragmatic. He will take things as they come and figure things out for himself. He also acknowledges a dark side that carries him in the opposite direction.

"I am not the happiest person in the world, but I still try to do the things I have always done. I believe that it is better to be upset and angry and do something, as opposed to being upset and angry at yourself and doing nothing." Ben's anger at himself sounded close to the self-loathing I experience when I fail at a physical task. My fault, I feel.

This certainly did not sound like acceptance. "No, it does not." And too frequently, Ben does not sound like a happy guy. Punishing ourselves for our physical flaws is an unfortunate side effect of having a disability.

Negotiating life's logistics long ago replaced dancing with the furies for the older Cumbos. For years, young Ben's everyday needs forced his family to anticipate and plan each day. But the time came for Ben to leave home, and the family was ready, even Ben. "Actually, I was scared as hell, but it was time," he said. Ben did not know anybody at St. Mary's College and knew that he would have to reestablish himself and work hard to feel as though he belonged.

"You can take care of yourself," I had told him before he left home. "You know that."

"It is important for Ben to see that," his dad had added, as the three of us sat in their living room one afternoon after Ben's high school graduation. "It will be no big thing," young Ben commented rather dismissively. He did not want to hear the lecture.

Still, departure would include high drama. Getting Benjamin Cumbo IV out of the house and off on his marvelous journey, building the future his doctors had suggested might not come, was only the beginning. Ben and Debi paused, at least momentarily, in satisfaction.

"We helped Ben navigate the waters. He has self-confidence and wants to live a normal, full life." That belief in himself would have to stick. "On good days, it is there," Dad said. The not-so-good moments would tell the tale.

Mom had her own issues and emotions. "Fear," she laughed uneasily. "There is a lot of fear involved." Whose? "Mine," Debi giggled. "Looking at him, knowing what it takes for him to navigate day to day, I worry," she admitted.

The self-confidence of a vulnerable guy would be measured first by a new routine. "Ben will have to go to the bathroom in the middle of the night. He might be alone and incapacitated." Then she cut to the chase. "I have a fear of humiliation for him. He has a ton of pride. To see him in a situation where he cannot help himself is what keeps me awake at night."

That was the shared fear that haunted mother and son. Debi was not afraid for Ben's life. "The threat is the little things that able-bodied people just take for granted." Those common crises could drop this young man in his tracks.

That warning became real during Ben's first semester at college. The college owned several townhouses that sat at a distance off the busy main road. These fancier digs were in demand among students and seemed to answer Ben's physical needs. But instead of the communal living experience of the dorm, Ben found himself in a small, isolated house with unknown and, it turned out, unreliable roommates.

Ben swallowed hard and told himself he was ready to reach out. "I probably will need to ask my roommates and other people if they can assist me with things," he had said before leaving for college. "I guess once I get to know other people for a day, that will be all the trust I basically need, in a sense, to think, Okay, this person seems cool enough for me. They do not seem upset or anything, so I can basically ask them for help anytime."

Then came the ambush. Ben's roommates were loud, disruptive, and ready to party. He had long ago decided to steer clear of alcohol because of his 24/7 need to keep his wits at close range. On one night, his roommates returned to the house from a night of partying. "They were drunk, really drunk," Ben recalled. They were raucous, the noise continuing until, one by one, they fell asleep.

Ben needed help getting on and off the toilet. Someone helped him that night for the ascent but he was abandoned for the descent. "I called out and waited. Finally, I gave up and crawled across the floor and into my room." There he lay, unable to get into bed without help.

"Ben called me. It must have been two or three in the morning," his dad said. "I tried calling the townhouse from my cell phone and got no answer. I was about to get into the car and drive for more than an hour down to the school just to get Ben into bed. I was upset for him." The young man called again. "No, Dad," Ben insisted. "I will just reach up and pull down a blanket and pillow, and I can sleep on the floor."

That was it. Young Ben had crossed the Rubicon. "I had decided, 'Enough.' In the bathroom, I thought, This is the last straw. I am not going to deal with this anymore." He went to the St. Mary's administration to ask for new roommates.

"There could have been a fire," Ben's father said. "These guys might not have heard the alarm and helped Ben out of there." The school officials acknowledged that they were not watching closely enough.

The Cumbos hired a health care professional to come to Ben's room each morning to help him bathe and dress. That a stranger would be doing for him what his Mom and Dad had done for his entire life bothered him terribly until he got used to it.

"Think of her the way you would a doctor," Dad had counseled. "There is no reason to be self-conscious."

The routine was as it had been at home. "I wake up, and the first thing I do is change. Then the ritual every morning is I put my braces on and then I have to put my pants on over that and my shoes." Ben could not complete that last phase of dressing alone.

Ben possesses the ability to see through himself and, however long it has taken, to deal with his own foibles. "In these situations, pride can get the best of you, to the point where you hurt yourself," he said quietly. "It takes a bigger man to admit that he needs help than to say he does not."

In dealing with the regular melodrama of my own

life, occasionally I indulge in the internal scream. Wait a minute, I shriek to myself. This is not how I want to live. Come on, this is not my life. Yeah, right. That lament *How did this happen to me?* is usually triggered by the small stuff that suddenly looms large.

"Do you ever ask that question?"

"Yes." Ben chuckled. "You are right. It is the insignificant things that make you want to scream out sometimes." We can wonder, but to no avail. "I wonder, but that does not give me an answer, so I do not think about it." Case closed.

Ben's ability to shut off debate, to silence the critic in his head, has to be useful. Those dark decrees can overpower the rational voice. They take you nowhere. The discipline and personal strength necessary to control the raging inferno in his head puts him more in control of himself. For him, as perhaps for so many, this sort of silencing is a defense mechanism, necessary to protect against not just unexpected events but his own emotions.

Planning for the failures of others, such as roommates, seems a tedious task. "I control myself and get irritated because I expect people to be grown up when they act like children." Ben has no time for that. "Self-reliance is standing up," he says emphatically.

MORE THAN ANYTHING, Ben needs to feel normal. A critical piece of that normalcy to him seems to be some serious, yet undefined relationship with a young woman. For a long time he has wanted to take those first steps. Just to talk. To sit together. To share.

So much of his anxiety about meeting and getting to

know members of the opposite sex stemmed from his xenophobia, the unshakable fear of others. Old fears die slowly. He was skittish about the rejection he expected would come.

"If I were to try to talk to a girl, I guess, I would think, Okay, she is not going to want to talk to me at all," he said gloomily. Not at all? "Maybe she is going to wonder what I am doing, trying to speak to her. It's stuff like that." His darkly pessimistic scenario took on a life of its own. "I can imagine, like, hundreds of people laughing at me if I try to say something." This fear of humiliation almost bordered on paranoia.

Erin said she had offered consistent advice to her brother about meeting members of the opposite sex. "'Get girls to be your friend,' I tell him. 'Stop looking at them like you have to holler at a girl all the time.'" Erin looked disapproving. "That is what his friends are doing," she added. "Those guys are making themselves look like idiots."

Ben's flirtation with black street culture, which he seemed to know little about, instructed him that coarse is cool. "That is not Ben," his father chuckled. "He has to find that out for himself."

Tyler had helped her older brother sort out the issue of relationships, which, of course, is a high priority for any teenager. She pointed out that she is closer in age to her brother than is Erin, and the two were able to compare notes on their social lives. "He is always asking me for advice, like, 'Should I call her? Should I instant-message her?' I tell him, 'Just be yourself. That is what people like about you.'"

For any teenager, the stakes are high. For a disabled teenager, the risks shoot through the roof. "For me, the

risk is rejection and how I will feel after I meet someone."
Ben admitted his tendency to hang back. "Yeah. I am
always hesitant to try to talk to girls," he explained. He,
or anybody in the sitting position and looking for a standup companion, could speak of growing self-confidence or
pride. Still, the plaintive cry was sounded.

"What is a poor guy like me doing, trying to meet girls?"
Then the self-recrimination began. "I am not normal. Not
everybody is going to want to be with me."

"How do you know?"

"I just do. People have no idea what it is like to be in
wheelchair." And he assumes the worst. "I will never know
if my failures are because I am disabled or just bad at talking."

Girls, the hope goes, will see something in this young
man whom they admire and will give him a shot. "People
who know me or my sisters will give me a fair chance. But I
will say that a disabled guy is not for everybody." You have
to keep trying. "There has to be some physical attraction
for them. I don't know," he trailed off.

BEN ROLLED INTO the kitchen in his reassigned digs. New
roommates wandered in and out. Ben came across as the
loner. Intense seriousness separates him from his peers. He
is on a mission to make a life. He will not be stopped. In
that darkened suite on campus, his nose stayed in a book.
"Eventually, I will come to terms with my situation and
accept."

He has a long way to go before he can say he has learned
to accept. Maybe resignation more than acceptance is where
young Ben's emotions take him. As he says, "This is my life,

and it may be unfortunate, but this is what I have to put up with. The only option I really have is to live with it."

He continued to frame the struggle according to his fears and his dealings with others. He works to put that fear of others to rest. "People are not always going to be nice to you, but I also started to realize that people are inherently good. Not everybody is out there to get me." I wasn't always sure that he believed his own words.

Older sister Erin believes that Ben will find it hard to change, that his negative thoughts cloud his judgment. "It is almost like Ben thinks he can hear people thinking about him, and that is just not true." Erin worries about her brother. "He has got these voices telling him what is going on." Those voices instruct Ben to watch out.

Erin's growing optimism about her new career as an urban planner is tempered by fears for her brother's future. "I pray that Ben just continues to grow," she said, "that nothing happens that is going to paralyze him so he does not want to go any further."

Ben struggles to control a shotgun distrust that sprays wide. That abiding suspicion of others has seemed to block his path to a relationship. "I think Ben is trying to prepare himself by assuming that when he gets into a situation, he is going to be hurt by it," Erin observed. "I say, 'When a person meets you, they can tell right away. You are just a nice guy to talk to.'"

Ben creates his own isolation, and then suffers from it. "Being alone is something I can deal with," Ben said as he pondered a solo future. We were alone in his darkened room at school. Ben turns his frustration away from muscular dystrophy and projects it on to others. That way people, not the disease, become the enemy. "I am angry, I guess. I'm sad." And worse, he feels humiliated. He has turned this humiliation on himself. "I am known to see myself as a loser, somebody who is unwanted." He is setting himself up to be alone.

Late one night, Ben called his sister Erin after returning to his townhouse from a mixer. In full frustration, the young man described the view from his wheelchair. "I am down here. Everyone else is standing up. They are talking about something up there, and I don't know what they are talking about," he recounted to his sister.

As Erin described it, Ben was beside himself. "I told him, 'Well, I am sure there are people who are sitting down. Not everyone is standing up. Not everyone is on the dance floor.'" Fear of someone standing, the dominant position, is an animal instinct.

A troubled mind frequently accompanies the battered body. Erin could feel her brother's emotional pain and wanted desperately to help him. "I said you have to figure out what is fun for you to do at a party." Erin believed her brother painted an unrealistic picture of parties in his head.

"I don't always dance when I am at a party," Erin said with her own frustration. "Sometimes, I am bored, hanging around and socializing. Ben sees the people who are sitting down as being the losers," she said. "He just categorizes everybody in the room as soon as he comes in."

Ben draws little comfort from the support around him, those who assure him he is not a loser. More than a few years into our relationship, I knew he was anything but. "People tell me constantly that it just is not the case," Ben agreed. Those reassuring words are not persuasive to him, however, and his dim view of himself can become a self-fulfilling prophecy.

Ben, in our many conversations, did seem determined to be unhappy. He cheerfully agreed that self-directed anger contributed to a pattern of low self-esteem. "Yeah. I get totally down on myself. I will admit I still do that, right up to now." On some level, we all succumb to self-slander, but some control it better than others.

"Maybe this is a matter of karma, guilt for sins of a former life."

"You are not serious."

"I am learning about reincarnation. It just might be."

"You got screwed, plain and simple," I said. "Get angry and get over it. Light the fire and let it burn through. You will feel better."

Ben applies what to me is a strange variation on the theme. "I have a weird philosophy," the young man said, "and I will sometimes beat myself up so that I will keep myself grounded, so I don't become too cocky and piss people off, I guess." That sounds like beating your head against a wall because it feels so good to stop.

Self-directed anger is another story. Turning the flame-thrower on yourself will burn a person beyond recognition. Facing the anger and acknowledging the humiliation that is the trigger can be painful for any suffering soul, perhaps an impossibility for a teenager. When my own humiliation grows intense, when I trip, stumble, and fall and there is nowhere to go with it, I, too, can turn fire on myself in frustration. Then I get over it, a clean burn. But Ben is too afraid of his anger to do anything but direct it against himself.

We were making our way across campus. The gentle hill down toward the river was flecked with snow and littered with fallen branches. I thought that maybe the bucolic surroundings would provide calm and help Ben lighten up.

Instead, he retreated into his hole once again. "It's just like Groundhog Day for the emotional stuff," he said. He did hold high hopes that he would continue to grow and change. "Maybe I will just go, Okay, that is tough. Get back up again. It's not so bad. You are still alive." That showed resilience, but the young man could not get himself to hold on to that positive perspective for very long.

Ben knows that his long war is waged against himself. Along the way, he is often disappointed in others. "People may not have a clear idea of what my life is or care."

"Do people owe it to you to care?"

"It does not hurt to know this stuff." The automatic response to upset too often is to lay blame at the feet of the other guy.

This young man does know the main battleground lies north of his own neck. That is where he must make his peace.

Ben understands that he has paid a steep price for his social panic. "I look out for trouble so much that I miss out on stuff that is really important, such as actually talking to people and enjoying myself." He recognized the dynamic even before finishing high school. Though his best intention is to grow, the pattern remains entrenched.

We had talked about this rut as students changed classes

at Bishop McNamara. As usual, Ben was moving alone. He rolled with me next to him to the tiny lift that would get him to the second floor. This was not an elevator but a hydraulic lift, specially constructed for Ben's use and installed in an empty space adjacent to the stairs.

We could not have traveled up that one floor together. The space on the lift was so confined that Ben alone would be making this short trip. Once again, he was pulled away from others, pushed into his own category. I watched him enter the lift, position the chair precisely. Back and forth he went, turning a little bit at a time.

The corridors were jammed with young people laughing and carousing, shouting their way to the next class. Ben was not part of that. He occasionally nodded to others but took his separate route, ever the solitary figure. He travels the road less taken because he must. The chair separates him from others. So does that fence he has constructed in his head. Don't you feel lonely?

"Sometimes," was all he would say about that on this day. I learned about another trauma visited on the Cumbo family, one that caused young Ben to feel less alone. After years of mysterious ailments, Debi was diagnosed with lupus, a serious autoimmune disease.

Lupus was one more family grenade to juggle. The Cumbos were maxing out. "We were losing control," Debi said. "We went through a period of practically shouting, 'Why us? Why now?'"

The challenge became how to turn the corner and leave high emotion behind. "You have to allow yourself to go through the other emotions to get over them," she said.

"Otherwise they fester. You have to cry and be angry and lash out." That means you think anger can be constructive.

"Yeah, I tell Ben all the time to get angry," she agreed. "But you cannot stay angry," she added. Therein lies the trap. "Sometimes I hold the anger in because, deep down, I am afraid I will go over the edge and not be able to come back."

Young Ben rode to the rescue. "Ben made me put my illness into perspective," Debi said. "I figured, if a child can do it, so can I." Then she went one step further, explaining that occasionally she switched roles with her son.

"Ben preached to me what I had preached for so long to him. 'Things are not that bad.' We talked a lot, and sometimes we cried together." Debi chuckled now. "It was good to have that kind of soul mate." Big Ben told me that his son had a strengthened sense of solidarity with his mom. "Now she had a disease, too. Ben was not alone."

Helping Mom had been a mission for her son. Young Ben had put anger aside for the moment. Controlling, not extinguishing the flame is the key. When a prominent New York psychiatrist learned that I had endured two bouts of colon cancer as well as multiple sclerosis, his response was direct: "You must have been in a rage" was his immediate comment over coffee. Well, good morning, doctor. The man did not speculate about frustration or depression. This shrink just headed to rage. Do not pass Go. Do not collect two hundred dollars. "Are you still angry?" he inquired. Yup. Anger is not abnormal.

Calm, too, can become a coping mechanism. For Debi and Big Ben, pouring water on the emotional fires was a way of buying time to steady themselves. "I am trained as a defense analyst not to lose my head," Big Ben explained. "I have learned to maintain control. That is how I find stability." Debi, too, learned to look before leaping into the fray.

Emotion must be released, however. Debi had a keen sense of when the time was right, and would push her husband to let go. "My wife prods, and then it does come out." Big Ben chuckled. "I weep, and we talk. We confess our fears to each other."

At the close of his freshman year, Ben learned that because of his book, he had been selected as an Emerging Artist for 2006 by the sorority Delta Sigma Theta. He was recognized at American University in Washington before a large audience. I reminded him that he had said long ago he wanted to be taken seriously as a writer. "Isn't that what is happening?"

"It seems that way," he answered a bit self-consciously. "It is happening quicker than I ever dreamed."

"Aren't you proud?"

"I know I should give myself some credit," he said almost grudgingly. "Maybe it is a mixture of pride and humility. I am a young African American male telling my story. Okay. I will say, I am proud."

"Thanks," I said back. "And I am proud of you."

THE WALL AROUND Ben stands tall, shutting even his family out. "Ben can keep even us at a distance," Debi said one evening. "Our son is very protective of his feelings." Tyler, only a few years younger, rose to the challenge of breaking through. Sometimes siblings know the best angle of engagement.

Tyler's effort came intuitively and was built on their long years together. "We always laughed together," she said. "We cracked jokes. If we had not been that close growing up, then I don't think we would be this close now. Now we talk every day on the Internet, or he calls just to talk to me."

Tyler describes a typical conversation. "'Ben, how do you feel?' 'Okay,' he will say. 'No, seriously, how do you really feel? What is going on?' I just kept at it with Ben."

Tyler laughed. "You have to really beat it out of him for him to tell you the truth. I think that is pretty normal, just the kind of person he is." Tyler and I were talking in the empty gym at Holy Cross Academy in suburban Maryland outside Washington. The young woman played serious basketball in this cavernous space.

This was Tyler's home court, her comfort zone. Tears flowed as she described her fierce desire to ease her brother's burden. The young athlete spoke of endless assaults on his dignity. "I told my mom that I wish I could take some of his pain away, because I never know how he really feels. You never know his true pain."

The hurt spread to the family as they watched Young Ben collapse into his wheelchair over time. "I know he is in pain when he cannot even help himself. You have to keep helping him all the time, knowing that he could not be alone."

Yet Ben showed no fear of being alone. "Do you worry about maybe not marrying in the future?"

"Somehow I think that is how my life is going to be," he told me. We were talking at the family house during a break from college. I flashed to a recent memory of Ben sitting alone in his wheelchair at the student center. He had looked like a lonely guy in a happy place, quietly eating supper as others in groups laughed and talked about their day.

"I may be a lonely person when I get older, because I am too scared to actually go outside my comfort zone and take a risk," he added. His dad was well aware that his son never had the luxury of taking risks. "If I have a regret for him," said Big Ben, "it is that he cannot take a chance, whether it is one that takes him to the edge of maybe changing his life or simply meeting a special person."

"I know this much," young Ben said. "Being alone is more sad than scary. If that is how it stays, I will be a really angry, bitter person, and who wants to be that for the rest of his life? Nobody does." This kid was under twenty when he said that, already girding himself against aloneness, the condition he possibly most feared.

The downside of living in your head is that when you free your demons, reality becomes irrelevant. Fantasy and fear combine to push any of us down a slippery slope, carrying us away from the reasoned view. Then we have to find our way home.

Ben and I sat amid the din of the student center, eating something I have yet to identify. "Like all things, you have to go through the storm a bit," Ben said almost casually. "I worry less and less because I am slowly learning not to be so pessimistic."

He pointed to lessons learned. "No matter how bad things may seem at any time, I have to try to make them work and just see." There came one more pause. "I can laugh at myself sometimes. I know. Things are not so bad. They can be pretty good."

* * *

CHILDREN'S HOSPITAL SITS atop another hill, this one in northwest Washington, a short ride up North Capitol Street from Union Station. The large hospital is a kid-friendly refuge for sick children.

A wide sunny three-story atrium is filled with traditional-looking hot-air balloons. Everything is colored in pastels. A puppet show in the lobby was playing to a smattering of children who were moving through various examining rooms and treatment areas. They sat in wheelchairs and hobbled on crutches and seemed genuinely happy for the diversion.

I was escorted into the muscular dystrophy command center, as the medical folks thumbing through the charts called it. This visit felt overdue. Young Ben's doctor walked into the area. She is an attractive, middle-aged woman with an infectious smile, animated and intense.

The doctor was born in Argentina. She lost no time in distancing herself from American medicine when the conversation turned to the quality of care. "A lot of the American way is with coldness, right?" She instantly won my vote. "It is as if I am going to treat you as a disease and not a person." Keep going.

We ducked into a vacant examination room to talk. My questions regarded Ben's or anyone's chances for achieving longevity with muscular dystrophy. "By the time they are in their wheelchairs, before they are twenty, usually they are dead. That is the natural history of the disease," the doctor said with obvious emotion.

She explained that early intervention with steroids was adding years to the lives of MD patients, that an additional ten to twenty years was not unusual. "Their respiratory function remains really good on the steroids, if you do not stop. So we have twenty-four-year-olds who have normal respiratory function. And there are people in their thirties who have jobs and lives with these steroids and other therapies. We have moved in the right direction with muscular dystrophy," she said, "but not far enough."

The doctor made plain that one's years are numbered by this disease. Of course, even for the healthy, life begins its slow end at first breath. "Yes, but muscular dystrophy is cruel and takes a life much earlier." She told me that losing young patients was increasingly difficult for her to endure. "I cannot go to funerals or viewings of my patients."

The doctor was unyielding and unequivocal. "There are a lot of people who go [to funerals]. I never did go, and I will not. I know I should be there. I feel very guilty that I do not go. But I just cannot." Suddenly I realized that the doctor was standing bolt upright, her back stiff and straight. "I do everything I can for them while they are here. I treat them aggressively. If they die, probably I will write a card or something." The doctor stopped in mid-thought. She appeared pained by the subject. "I only do well helping them while they are still alive." If death is a part of life, even the doctor, unable to heal her patient, searches for closure and struggles to find her own peace.

For this doctor, there is no such thing as acceptance. I asked Big Ben if he had accepted the situation. "Acceptance?" he threw back at me. He was almost challenging. "I think acceptance is a crock," he said with power in his calm voice. "People accept at the last moments of their lives." The man had thought this through. "We do not accept," he emphasized. "We are a family built and sustained on hope. That is our mantra."

Big Ben is too preoccupied with keeping his son going to entertain thoughts of acceptance. His strategic role with young Ben is to hold him on an even keel and keep hope going. "I cannot allow myself to get depressed along with him. I have to pump him up. That is critical."

The whole issue of acceptance haunts the sick and those who love and care for them. But what does making peace with an illness, finding this mythical, magical acceptance, even mean?

If this sounds like a word game, it is not. "Peace" and "acceptance" become vague concepts thrown around without enough thought. For the religious, acceptance can mean affirming orthodoxy. Our fate is God's will. I think of acceptance as giving in.

Of course we, the sick, accept a diagnosis. It is what it is, and we must move forward. Learning to focus on living is another matter. Ben understands at a very young age that he needs to determine the essence of who he is and where his dreams might take him. "I need to be able to focus on things that are real in life," he said, "and look at what I am and where I might be going."

This kid had guts. In the end, the whole Cumbo family demonstrates on a daily basis that they, too, have guts. They are living their lives to the fullest, keeping the faith and waiting for help. Debi sounded an optimistic note in that muscular dystrophy video a decade ago. "The doctors are working very hard to get this cure. They are so very close. One day soon, it is going to come."

Still, hope cannot wash away fear and pain. There can

be nothing more wrenching for any parent than helplessly watching a disease play out in a son or daughter of any age. "It is seeing a young person you love so much going through the emotional pain that you cannot take away or do anything about," Ben's dad told me, his own emotions frayed.

Finally, the two of us had wandered into the danger zone. We had touched on the uncomfortable conversation about young Ben's early mortality. We were sitting in the Cumbos' comfortable suburban Maryland home on a hot afternoon, sipping ice water at the kitchen table. I began hesitantly, forever fiddling with a tape recorder that never seemed to work when I needed it. The beast was hovering.

"Man, that is the toughest thing in the world, trying to bring yourself to face reality . . ." His voice cracked. "I think it is a tough job, trying to find peace."

"It must be a journey without end," I said softly.

"Oh, no question," Ben responded immediately.

"The biggest fear I have is, the biggest fear I ever had is," Ben said again, "that I will have to bury my son." He began to weep. "I would have that fear anyway, if there were not a disease. But this could happen." We sat looking at each other. "Richard, I want my son to bury his father."

On the muscular dystrophy video more than eight years earlier, a younger father expressed his grief. "You want initially to beat yourself up. You want it to just go away. You want to wake up because it is the most horrible nightmare you have ever had."

In his living room these many years later, Big Ben was

even more emotional. "I cannot . . . I just cannot bear to face that. I know that people die in wars. Kids can get hit by a car. But that is the chance we all take."

"Do you take satisfaction that you are doing everything you can for Ben, that he has the best care available?"

"Not really. I am the breadwinner. I am the protector of the family." Big Ben breathed deeply. "I failed. I did not protect. I did not do what was necessary to ensure that this did not happen." Big Ben, as with Buzz, feels a deep failure in his role as a traditional father.

My final meeting with the senior Cumbos came one summer afternoon at the University of Pennsylvania, where Tyler was attending basketball camp. Debi and Big Ben knew what I had come from New York to talk about.

The campus was quiet on this Saturday. We ambled past Franklin Field, named for a different Ben, and headed into the gym, The Palestra, with its rounded high ceiling and old iron girders.

We needed to have one last conversation about the contest young Ben would likely lose one day. "We are all going to die," Debi said quietly from a seat up toward the rafters. An athletic arena seemed an odd venue for this conversation. Basketballs pounding into the old wooden floor echoed throughout the empty gallery.

By now, the subject of death seemed strangely comfortable. "Some of us will die earlier than others. We do not know when. We do not know how," Debi began. "I could die before you do."

"Does young Ben get it?"

"Sometimes." Debi chuckled. "If we do not have control over it, why worry about it? It's not for me to say," she offered calmly, trailing off for a moment. "The man up-stairs does."

Big Ben had described his role keeping young Ben's spir-its up. Debi seems to understand that to keep her son even, she, too, must stay steady. "I have meltdowns," she admit-ted. And? Debi clenched the muscles in her jaw. "You boo-hoo. You beat the sheets. You beat the pillow," she said, hitting her leg emphatically with a fist. "You ask, 'Why, why, why?' Then, okay, it's done."

The next step puts the family back on track. "Now we have to move on. You must move forward."

"I guess you have no choice."

"Right. You can curse God," she said calmly, "but I cannot curl up into a ball and not deal with it. That is what we try to get Ben to see."

"When all is said and done," I said, "attitude will take a person only so far." The odds were against young Ben.

"Oh, yeah," his father responded quickly. "Yes, yes," echoed Debi.

"Does young Ben understand that?"

"I think that deep within himself he understands," Big Ben answered. "I think that haunts him."

We watched Tyler taking control on the basketball court below. The teenager was agile and fast on her feet, hitting long shots and driving to the basket. She was taking risks. Her physical prowess stood in stark contrast to her brother. Tyler has the family quota of self-confidence. The young woman seemed fearless.

"Ben would never share with us his true fears," his mom said as we sat in the stands. "He would not open up his feelings about what is to come."

"But he is a bright kid," I said.

Debi sat back and smiled. "Oh, he is." She stopped momentarily. "He has to know—"

Big Ben interrupted. "We hold on to hope. Hope is fleeting, but at the same time, we do not know. No one does."

The three of us were about the only folks left in the stands. The Penn women's basketball coach had walked over to the Cumbos to chat about Tyler. Her parents were glowing, pleased and proud. Tyler's tomorrows look bright.

Young Ben does not worry about what may happen tomorrow. "Ben lives for today," Big Ben said. "His accomplishments are for today. His world is today."

"How do I approach young Ben about tomorrow and the ticking clock?" I asked the Cumbos on that warm afternoon in Philadelphia. I felt uncomfortable at the prospect of even touching on the subject with their son.

"Let him see the difficulty you feel asking the question," Dad advised. "Be honest with him." Big Ben reassured me that honesty is a commodity his son values. "Ben is a noble guy." Big Ben was telling me that his son would rise to the occasion. "Ben can help you ask the questions, and that may help him answer."

Big Ben had carried his special calm into the gym. "Just like you have sat here with us and said you do not know how you are going to make him comfortable with it. I think you can ask him. I feel as his father that it is something he will address."

I did call Ben the following week. The Cumbos had told me he was ready to venture onto Washington's metro system and meet in the nation's capital. We picked a time and a place. Amtrak from New York was late. And I did not want to keep young Ben waiting, though Tyler was coming with him for an added sense of security.

The platform area at Union Station was stifling, brutally hot and awash in humidity as passengers disembarked. When I came up from the metro at the appointed station, there were crowds and traffic and street signs that were a blur for me, unreadable at any distance.

As I stumbled along the busy sidewalk, a young woman's voice rang out behind me. "Hey, Mr. Cohen," came the yell.

"Tyler," I said, "funny running into you here." Actually, I was grateful that they were a little late, too. Tyler was with a friend, and Ben rode along next to them. The young man sat jauntily in his chair, cap pointing backward.

There was the perfunctory and slightly awkward small talk. Ben gestured to his left. Across the teeming intersection sat a Barnes & Noble with the usual café upstairs. We had agreed on that spot for our rendezvous. Ben suddenly zoomed into the street through a curb cut before I could use my cane to negotiate a more significant step down.

Ben was wasting no time, cutting in front of turning vehicles, challenging buses and cabs, as if daring these predators to make a run at him. The kid certainly seemed sure of himself. This was not the tentative kid I had met when he was in high school.

We settled in the café. I wanted a coffee and turned to Ben. "What can I get you?"

"Nothing really," he answered.

"It is hot out there," I pointed outside. "Do you want a bottle of water?"

"Not really," Ben repeated. "I am fine." It occurred to me that he was reticent to take in fluids because he had no interest in negotiating the unseen bathroom in this strange place. As with Denise, he was eyeing the landscape and planning ahead.

"What have you learned from a year away from home?" I began.

"I have learned not to be a hermit but to put myself out there more," he answered, projecting a new confidence. Would he have come here to meet me a year ago? I asked. Ben smiled and laughed. "Probably not."

"Would you have taken a bus to the train and headed for Washington?"

"Prior to college, that would not have happened at all. I do not think I had the confidence to know I could do that stuff for myself."

Tyler and her girlfriend had wandered away, though I continued to feel their gaze from behind a stack of books somewhere. Customers came and went around us, paying little attention to the two guys and a tape recorder. My delaying tactics had run out.

"Are you afraid to die?" I finally asked.

There was not even a pause. "Not really," Ben answered quickly. "It is inevitable for all of us. There is no sense in being afraid of something that is inevitable." He laughed. "Just please do not tell me the date." That seemed reasonable.

"Is dying something you think about?"

"Oh, yeah, it is something I think about. What if there is nothing on the other side and this is it? Would I have wasted my life and I will just fade away?" Ben raised doubts about his Maker's job performance. "I certainly wonder why, if God is a magnificent being, why doesn't he get rid of the disease right now?" I hoped he was not expecting an answer.

"Ben, do you want something to eat?" I was thinking I would rather hear this kid chew than listen to him talk about dying.

"No, thanks. I am good."

"Ben, we have gone back and forth about religion. How important is it in coping with your illness?"

"To be honest, organized religion just gets on my nerves. Every religion says we are going to heaven, and everyone else is going to hell. I cannot believe that."

"What do you believe?"

"Whether you call God Allah, Jahveh, whatever you believe God's name is, or if you do not believe in God at all, everyone finds their way. I do not believe in politicizing something that spiritual and close to your heart." Doubt spoke for itself.

"If you are looking for religion to fix all your problems, it is not going to get you anywhere," Ben answered. "I believe that God will not help us if we have the strength in ourselves to do it. It is only at that time when we just cannot do it that divine intervention comes in."

This young man seems to believe in the burden of personal responsibility. The Lord, it seems, is not his co-pilot. "I believe it is up to us to make a difference in our own lives. I think we have a core of strength we can rely on in tough situations." Only a kid with a life-threatening disease or bullets whistling overhead thinks through these highly personal questions at this age.

Then how do you do it? I came close to demanding. What is the magic?

"I knocked some sense into myself, knowing that I am in a tough situation," Ben answered calmly. "There are billions of people in this world who live a lot worse than I do. There are people who are starving and do not have anything."

"But you are an endangered species. This is your life. You might die sooner than you expect. Is the relative plight of others enough to get you through?"

"I could be a soldier in Iraq right now, and God bless those guys. That helps quell my frustration. My gratitude takes over. I have a loving family and a roof over my head. It may not be a cure-all, but my selfishness can fade away and I realize how lucky I am, how blessed I am."

I blinked hard. "And you mean it when you say you are lucky."

Ben sat back and smiled. Actually, he grinned. I think he had figured out that the conversation was coming to a close.

"Thank you, Ben," I said as I reached for his hand. "This was hard work, and you are a trooper to talk with me."

"This was good," Ben said suddenly. "You forced me to think about stuff." Already, he seemed to be evaluating our ad hoc relationship. Our intense dialogue and budding friendship had evolved.

Ben understands that his journey will be cut short. As with Denise and Buzz, the ticking is loud, the days numbered. And he is barely twenty, old beyond his years. Some chronic illnesses bring inevitability into a life. There will be no appeal.

Tyler and her buddy appeared on cue for our goodbyes. In the end, Ben had looked hard into his life, discovering no greater peace than he could claim as we began our dialogue. With whom, if I may ask, should he have made that peace? Perhaps his Maker? His mother? Himself? Any of those would make sense, Ben would agree.

I looked into Ben's eyes and could see the wheels slowly turning. That movement never ceases. "I promised your mom you would be on the train before rush hour. You should get going."

"Don't worry about me." Ben chuckled. "I have plenty of time," he said with no hint of irony. And the three were on their way, vanishing into the elevator.

Reflections

Valuing Quality Over Quantity

Our journey toward death begins at birth. Yet acknowledgment and acceptance of mortality do not kick in until we are far down the road. Time seems to stand still when we are young. We see ourselves as indestructible.

This youthful bravado was knocked out of Ben long ago. His life may be more than half over as he enters his twenties. My experience with illnesses prompts me to look at my life and ask, How hard the journey? Ben can only wonder, how short?

A death-dealing illness forced Ben to grow up and confront the meaning of an abbreviated life. Yet he seems not to hear a clock ticking on his time here. Instead of self-pity or fear, he embodies ambition and a sense that there are no limitations. Opportunity and careers are what occupy his thoughts. His recent internship with Sen. Barack Obama was an exciting step, a new beginning on his uncertain path. Ben fixes on the contours of the road ahead, not its length. There is too much work to be done, perhaps no time to waste. His refusal to play victim seems instinctive. He dares to dream.

He has no idea how strong he is, how fierce his optimism, how powerful his selective denial. He is a living example of what I've come to believe: denial is liberating because it throws off despair and makes all things possible in the time we are given. Ben teaches us that adding quality to a life is all that matters; not its length. The "what ifs" and "one days" disappear in pursuit of the now, and life has new meaning.

five

Sarah Levin

Seeking Normalcy

SARAH LEVIN AND I shook hands at the airport, meeting for the first time. We stood outside the terminal, taking stock of each other as we made small talk. Then the two of us headed out, picking up coffees and driving into Cleveland. I watched intently, focusing on Sarah behind the wheel as she tooled along the highway into the city.

We were going across town to her office in Shaker Heights, passing close to some of Cleveland's tougher areas. We left the highway so that Sarah could show me around. There was a reason for the quick tour. This young woman wanted me to see who she is and where she spends much of her days.

Sarah is a social worker who works with kids from the city's poorest neighborhoods. Our trip now was taking us through some dicey districts. "As long as we are here," she

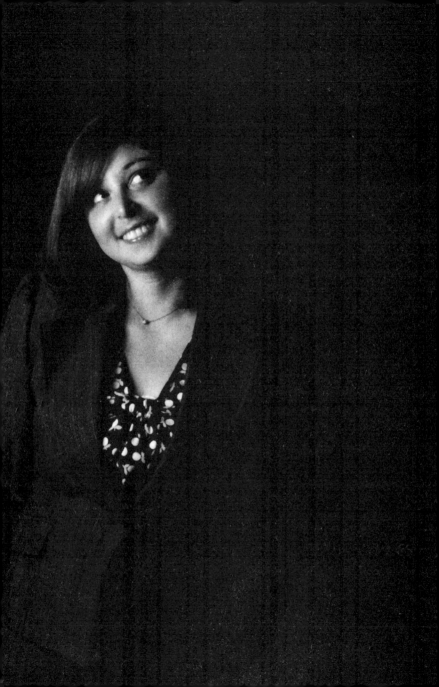

said, "I need to pick something up. It will save me a trip later."

We pulled into a driveway in front of a house that had seen better days. Sarah needed to get a document from a client. I waited in the front seat, watching this small woman approach the silent house. The old wooden structure seemed foreboding, the neighborhood rough.

When no one answered the door, Sarah walked back past the car, holding up one finger, signaling, "Be back in one minute." She seemed unbothered by where she stood, though this did not feel like a welcoming place. She disappeared around back and vanished. She has guts, I thought. She reappeared, papers in hand.

Sarah counsels troubled kids and their families at an experimental school that draws children from around the city. I had spent enough time in Cleveland during my years in the news business to remember journalists mocking the worn place as The Mistake on the Lake. A brief urban resurgence had given way to the feel of a Rust Belt town that could not keep up with a new era.

Sarah seemed to be smaller than life, a pretty version of Stuart Little's kid sister, diminutive and always on the go. The two of us walked and talked, jumping or, in my case, stumbling back into the car to drive through more projects in areas Stuart would never choose to visit. Sarah seemed so small up against this urban wasteland with its big problems.

She described going into broken homes and dealing with hostile people, many of whom live with crack vials and cracked dreams. Troubled kids from that world can end up at Sarah's school and in her life. "My friends ask, 'Doesn't it scare you to go into these projects and take chances to do your work?'" Sarah carries pepper spray when she remembers to, in case she is attacked. "Nobody bothers me," she said. "I have been nervous at times but never really fearful for my life."

There is another threat that she does take seriously. Sarah suffers from Crohn's disease. She has a particularly bad case of that debilitating condition of the digestive tract. Crohn's wreaks havoc continuously on Sarah's already damaged body, creating daily doubts about her future.

Sarah pulled her red Volvo into the Fair Hill Center on the border of Cleveland and Shaker Heights on this steamy early afternoon. The July heat was oppressive, and the prospect of abandoning our air-conditioned cocoon, even for a short stay at her office, was unappealing.

Sarah looked fragile and walked slowly. "I am working just three days a week this summer," she explained as we headed toward the office and our next breath of cold air. "I just cannot do anymore," she said, "at least not right now." She juggles sickness and her social work, and the two are not easy companions.

This inflammatory bowel disease compromises Sarah's life each day. She seems exhausted beyond her twenty-eight years, as her soft, sometimes shaky voice betrays. "It is good," she said softly, "when there is more time to sleep. I sleep a lot these days. I think a lot of the fatigue comes from the fact that I am always anemic."

Chronic exhaustion is a byproduct of continual bleeding. Sarah had to have her large intestine removed, and the remaining upper digestive tract is so ravaged, it regularly hemorrhages into her belly. Bleeding is slow but steady, the blood working its way south to become rectal bleeding. "Internal, external, let's just say bleeding," Sarah said wearily.

She can speak openly without opening up in detail. Although she is a rock in her professional identity, she is uncertain socially and as a woman. This is not surprising; young women do not share the intimate specifics of intestinal misery with guys so easily. So Sarah lives as different people, one a shrinking presence, the other an expansive personality. A real-life incarnation of the Pushmepullyou, Dr. Dolittle's mythical animal tugging in opposing directions from itself, her vulnerability vies with her resolve. "I am more the tough person who has days of being vulnerable," she said. "Yeah, I do stand up in my life," she exclaimed as if surprised by her words.

Today, the old Fair Hill buildings house adult daycare facilities, serving seniors who do not need nursing homes but require stimulation and supervision during the day, as well as the school program where Sarah works. The dignified old place used to house a mental institution. "It seems appropriate," Sarah told me. Why? "My life is nuts," she answered with a half-smile and left it at that.

As an in-school therapist, Sarah works in and outside the classroom with kids who have trouble wielding social skills. Her program is called intergenerational because teachers and counselors work with the seniors at the center together with the kids. Some of the youngsters have behavioral problems. "I am there to intervene and work with parents."

"Does your career choice have anything to do with your health?"

"I went into social work because, eventually, I want to work with kids with colitis and Crohn's."

I watched Sarah out of the corner of my eye as we ambled down the school's long corridors. She has a grown-up mission but cannot shake her little girl look. She is tiny, standing just short of five feet on a good day. Her face is round and pink. Her physical stature is an unhappy by-product of imperiled health and pharmaceutical therapies for her disease. Drugs have resculpted if not deformed her body. And they have kept her alive.

By measures that go beyond inches, Sarah seems small in spirit. Wherever and whenever we have met, she has seemed solid as a survivor but tired from the steep vertical climb the sick must endure to reach their last stop, normal-cy. Her journey has been under way since childhood.

SARAH LEVIN HOLDS no memories of a carefree child-hood. In some real ways, she never knew the luxury of being a kid. As child turned toddler, adolescent turned adult, she was too busy straining to get through the day.

Sarah was barely out of diapers when the war with her body broke out. She was only three when the bloody diar-rhea began. The problem quickly escalated. "My parents have told me I was pretty much sick most of the time," she said.

Sarah's earliest memory of dealing with the illness was undergoing her first colonoscopy, at the tender age of four. "Yeah, I was very unhappy to be in the hospital," she re-called. "I was pretty scared and confused." I remember my own horror at this un-fun procedure as an adult. I told Sarah I had been fifty. She laughed. "I got a Cabbage Patch doll for agreeing to do it without a struggle. What did you get?"

"A headache," I answered.

Following the colonoscopy, Sarah was diagnosed with ulcerative colitis, a chronic inflammation of the colon that produces ulcers and pockets in its lining. The condition can produce intense abdominal pain, cramps, and loose discharges of pus or blood and mucus from the bowel.

That was the beginning of a long pattern of being sick and missing school. The hemorrhaging got worse. "I think I was in second grade when I got really sick," Sarah said. "I probably should have been hospitalized at that point." When she returned to school, her mother, Joan, went with her. "I cannot believe she did this," Sarah said, "but she would sit in the hallway all day." Joan spent hours reading, at the ready in case Sarah got sick. "I was there for weeks," Joan said.

Joan is an elementary school art teacher who was as concerned for Sarah's head as for her body. "The issue was insecurity on Sarah's part," Joan explained. "She was embarrassed, running to the girl's room, trying to make it before she got sick. The disruption usually came in the morning."

The problem was that Sarah was taking oral steroids. The little girl was swallowing prednisone to calm her gut. As an unwelcome side effect, the steroid also took over the functioning of her adrenal gland. That, in turn, left Sarah terribly nauseated after she awakened, virtually every morning.

Sarah's public vomiting was unpredictable, whether it was at a friend's house or on the camp bus. "I sat in that hallway because Sarah did not want to be sick in front of her classmates," Joan said. "She was so self-conscious."

A hovering mother at school only accentuated Sarah's sense of existing in a separate universe from the rest of the kids. Nothing is worse for a kid than being different. "By then, I felt like I was not the same, and I think the other kids probably thought I was strange."

The kids were merciless. Why is her mom here? Can't she go to school by herself? "At that point, I was not able to explain to other people what was wrong with me or what disease I had." Sarah makes it clear she did not understand her own problems. "All I knew, really, was I had tummy problems. If somebody did ask me, I would say, 'I have a bad tummy.' I did not know more than that, certainly nothing about ulcerative colitis."

There can be no memory, no precise fix on the moment of realization of serious sickness in an innocent child. It's not as though Sarah woke up one morning and understood that she was different or that her future was in doubt. The process of awakening to the realization that her illness would be forever happened gradually and over time.

"It was instinct," Sarah observed. "No one said anything about it to me." She remembers no particular emotion. "I was not emotional about my illness when I was younger. I just had it. That's all."

Sarah's childhood continued to be punctuated with frequent bouts of rectal bleeding and continual diarrhea. The discomfort, sometimes graduating to pain, became a defining piece of her young identity. "I would not be able to make it through the day without going to the nurse with a terrible stomachache."

"It all kept happening, and I felt more and more different," Sarah told me with no discernible emotion. "I just could not seem to get over it. I just knew that I was not like my friends. I do not think I knew how I was different, but I knew that I was different," she remembered. "I had the experiences with kids asking me why my face was so round, which was from the steroids."

Sarah's identity of being different took hold, exacting its toll. Kids made fun of her, as only kids can. "I have this vivid memory; I think I was six years old, and I was in our skating club and I remember a little boy. He asked a bunch of questions. 'Why is your face so round? Why are you so little? Why are you always on the end of the line in the skating shows?'"

These blunt inquiries marked the first time other children would point out that Sarah was different. "I guess I really did not know at that moment that my face was round because of the steroids." Sarah said her parents did what they could to shield her, but there's no way for a child to understand the difference between the innocent curiosity of another child and the hurtful comments of a bully.

Mom described the insensitive remarks of other parents who would ask blunt questions: "What is wrong with Sarah? Her face is so round." All the finger-pointing bothered Sarah a lot. "I just did not know why I had to be different." That became her lament, a recurring theme of Sarah's song.

She looked away thoughtfully, as if staring at something over my shoulder. "'Different' really is the word," she continued. "It made me sad, but the feeling that I was not the same stayed with me." Sickness can be a lonely experience.

"I was trying to feel that I did fit in, but the remarks felt like a slap in the face."

As adults, some of us celebrate our differences. For a kid, nothing matters more than fitting in and drawing little attention as an individual. Sarah was getting noticed, and for all the wrong reasons.

Her mother and her father, Paul, were determined that Sarah lead a successful life. Such a strategy can guide an ill youngster through the minefields of childhood. "My parents never let me feel sorry for myself," Sarah said. "They tried to do whatever they could to not make me feel like a victim. That was not an option. I am telling you, I was pushed into activities."

Debi and Ben Cumbo fought the identical battle with young Ben a decade later. Keeping youngsters strong in spirit and facing forward is a piece of the struggle when illness comes to kids. Youth get sidetracked as other kids become the issue, replacing illness as the enemy. Kids relate to one another, not to microbes and viruses.

Sarah figure-skated, took up ballet, played the violin. She became a Brownie, then a Girl Scout. "Yeah. I did everything that my friends were doing, and my parents made it a point for me to be involved in as many things as possible."

Of course, that particular approach to coping can become its own tyranny. "I was probably involved in more things than the average young child." Mom was the driving force. Joan did suggest and push, though she encountered little resistance. "These were all things I wanted to do," Sarah said.

Joan and Paul say with certainty that the battle became

as much psychological as physical. Sarah needed to know that her life was all about what she still could do. The couple seemed as sensitive to what went on in Sarah's head as in her gut.

At a 1998 luncheon for women of distinction in Cleveland, the Crohn's and Colitis Foundation honored Joan Levin for making a difference in the life of a child. Joan quoted the powerful advice she received long ago from Sarah's doctor: "You can take your daughter home and raise her with a sick child mentality, or you can raise her as a normal child, expecting from her what you would from any healthy little girl."

Sarah's dad, an attorney now serving as assistant law director for Beachwood, Ohio, a neighboring town, says, "My approach to treating Sarah normally probably was much more subtle than Joan's was. Joan tended to hit things head on." Paul's style was more laid back. He was inclined to step away and let events unfold. "I just figured, you want to do ice skating, all right, skate. Play your music. I was never willing to think of Sarah as unable to do, that we had to push."

The plan worked, but Dad still worries that Sarah may have misread signals. "Sarah may have felt I was ignoring her and downplaying real problems," Paul said. "But Sarah did come through."

Sarah's parents set the bar high and expected the best from their child. "I agree," Sarah said quickly. "I think that being able to participate in all those things, and my parents choosing not to allow me to stay home and moan because I had a stomachache, was the best thing that they did for me. I mean, that is why I am who I am today."

The unanswerable question is whether a person diagnosed in childhood adjusts well because there is no basis for comparison. Sarah never knew good health, so, like Ben, she can't miss what she never had. I, on the other hand, learned that I had multiple sclerosis when I was twenty-five and had enjoyed a normal life until then. For me, the shock of hearing such an awful diagnosis has stayed with me.

"Really, I started figuring out more about my problems at six or seven," Sarah said slowly. "It was not as if a light-bulb went off." Sarah just stopped. "I do not think my parents or doctors ever sat me down. I somehow developed this understanding myself."

Sarah remembered looking through books, though not absorbing much about ulcerative colitis. She seemed to develop a sixth sense or overheard conversations about the disease.

"I think we addressed the problems as they occurred," Joan said. "We just intuitively decided what was the right thing to say." She thought for a moment. "We never sat down and said, just, 'This is what you have, this is what you are in for.'" Joan assumed Sarah heard the term "ulcerative colitis" from doctors during casual conversations. "Things were discussed in front of her." Growing up with an illness, with or without a name that means anything, probably did ease Sarah into the tough realities she will live with for the rest of her life. There may be a wrong way to tell a young child about a sickness. Probably there is no right way. "It happened slowly, but we did not dwell on my health."

FOR SARAH, THE hardest part of dealing with disease has been taking the steroid prednisone on a regular basis.

The drug of choice for treating irritable bowel diseases, prednisone has a wide range of side effects. I have taken the pharmaceutical a number of times, and all it did was make me fat and crazy. Ben, too, took the drug with some benefit and harm: it helped preserve his lung function but also retarded his growth.

We who suffer from a range of chronic or autoimmune illnesses can become captives of a tyranny of treatment. The drugs we must swallow, the needles we thrust into our arms and legs, come with a price. These wonder drugs can bring on reactions that make us wonder why we are doing this to ourselves in the first place.

For Sarah, prednisone became a daily ritual at age four. "My mom mushed it into apple sauce." The drug has created a spectacular struggle for Sarah. It most likely has saved her life, but it has stunted her growth and softened her bones. And she has suffered unwanted weight gain on top of everything else.

As a teenager, Sarah suddenly began experiencing wild mood swings. "In the middle of a conversation, just one word or glance would cause me to burst into tears or jump down someone's throat," she said. Prednisone can make a person hypersensitive, a condition already common in adolescent girls.

Sarah was slow to connect the drug to her volatile feelings. "I knew about the other side effects," she said, "but for years I just thought I was really messed up." Joan, too, was stumped. "I attributed the mood swings, the ups and downs, to be about teenage girls and their mothers."

One unresolved question for Sarah and her family is to what extent prednisone has masked her true identity.

Powerful drugs do alter personalities and change behavior. "We do not know Sarah's real personality because she was on steroids for so long, really from a toddler on," Joan said. "How are we going to sort that out?" She sighed. "I wonder if we will ever know the real Sarah."

For teenage Sarah, the hot-button issue was her looks. Teenage girls are particularly obsessed with their appearance, and not surprisingly, remarks about her distorted face and body "made me feel so alienated."

Sarah switched drugs for a while. The new pharmaceutical was termed a steroid-sparing drug, intended to counter difficult side effects. But along came a new one. "I took the drug for a while but got horrible acne. It was a very big thing," Sarah said. "I never had pimples before. Here was yet another crisis to deal with. For a while, my skin was all I thought about."

Before too long, the prednisone was back. Sarah felt beleaguered and over time invented a dangerous game. She tried to fine-tune how much prednisone she had to swallow each day to get by. She was desperate to reduce the side effects, the moon face and weight gain that were psychologically so damaging.

The desperate move backfired, and Sarah found herself in the emergency room. The pattern continued, taking her to the hospital five or six times for extreme fatigue, dehydration, and increased bleeding. The sequence of crises was exhausting. Sarah was so weakened she could not pull herself out of bed. "Emotionally, it was terrible. I knew what I had done, and my body was out of control. I was a complete mess."

Sarah remembers this time as being utterly devastating. "I was a mess because I knew I would be put on even heavier doses of steroids in the hospital, and the side effects were going to rear their ugly head. That was inevitable."

"This was a self-inflicted wound."

"To some extent, yes," Sarah responded in a weary voice. "I think a saner person would have figured out how to find a happy medium. You either feel good or look good. A really sane person would have opted for feeling good," she concluded. Then her voice went up a notch. "Side effects are so damaging. They are so ugly," she added with a touch of the sullen. "Put yourself in my position."

Common sense prevailed, and Sarah relented. The prednisone cycle was resumed and is now kept intact. Sarah does dance close to the edge but more carefully. "I finally know how to gauge it so I am about a week away from landing in the hospital," she said, laughing. "I do wonder if ultimately the drug is worse than the disease," she said. "It just might be. Honestly, I have tried to figure that out. I think about it, sometimes every day." The question is difficult because pros and cons are extreme. Life without the drug might pay off for a while, with a patient looking better, that is, before the nosedive begins and picks up speed, putting the person in extreme danger.

That someone so young has had to build a life around a debilitating disease and powerful drug is cruel. And prednisone is the tip of the iceberg. "I take," Sarah began, trailing off. "I take," she repeated haltingly. "I take," pausing once more and staring into the distance as she lifted fingers.

She began to reel off names of drugs. There were pills for pain, drugs for diarrhea; Cipro, which she has taken for six years because she is prone to infection; another antibiotic that she was worried about staying on for too long; Nexium, for acid reflux; drugs for depression. There were a few odds and ends, and then Sarah finished her list. "Oh," she said, adding one more pharmaceutical. "I take something for nausea," she said, naming something else unpronounceable.

"All told, how many pills do you swallow each day?"

"Hold on," she replied. "Let me calculate this." I waited patiently. "Eighteen pills a day." Eighteen? "Eighteen. Eighteen pills every day."

"Do you take them in one feeding?"

"No." She laughed. "I take some in the morning, and in the evening, some before bed."

"Every day?"

"Every day." Sarah's point about feeling different was sinking in.

I know the drill. For eight long years, self-administered injections ruled my life. Sometimes once per week, others three times in the same period. Some MS patients needle themselves every day. For me, pain or the discomfort were not the deal breakers. Only the rigidity of the ritual got to me. I had to do it. How strange to feel pleasure that the drugs appeared not to make a difference. That meant the stabbing could stop.

The state of siege inflicted by illness and drugs never ends. Always there is the awful question, What's next? Whatever the answer, and always there is a *next,* fatalism hovers nearby. Things always can get worse.

* * *

WHEN SARAH WAS fifteen, she developed what is called toxic mega-colon. The sound of that condition was ominous. "Like, my colon just blew up."

"You mean it ruptured?"

"No. It ballooned and there were out-pouches. It was very painful. I was really sick." She was hospitalized and released in May 1995, the day before her sixteenth birthday party, which she almost missed. That summer was horrendous. Again, Sarah was taking high doses of steroids, with predictable results.

"I was very, very unhappy, and knew that people were looking at me and thinking that something was not right." As always, reactions of others determined the measure of Sarah's health in her own eyes. "I remember going back to school for my junior year, and a girl I was friends with said to me when she saw me, 'Oh my God, what happened to your face?' I was like, who says things like that? This was a miserable time."

Sarah's condition deteriorated. She was sick for much of the following summer. Serious problems just kept coming. She was bleeding and bloated and black about the future. "I was pretty miserable." Unlike Job, Sarah was about ready to say enough.

"We did not say that out loud. The doctor said it for us." Sarah's doctors began the drumbeat, broaching the idea of surgery. You mean surgically removing your colon, the large intestine. "Yes. My colon was now badly malformed. It was free-floating and twisting. The long and windy digestive road was not tacked down anymore, as the doctors call a secure and stable colon."

The plan would entail a two-part surgery. The first would be to remove the colon and do a temporary ileostomy, allowing the base of the colon to heal. That would mean Sarah would have a bag, the plastic receptacle for waste delivered directly through the wall of the abdomen. Later, a second surgery would reverse the ileostomy.

This was all too familiar. I had undergone the same procedure when I had my second bout of colon cancer. This procedure was not fun, the bags, hideous. Cancer is no fun. Neither are diseases of the bowel. The Levins had run out of alternatives.

Sarah's parents took her to the Cleveland Clinic. The family sat with doctors to discuss the possible surgery. Sarah was seventeen now, young to be promoted to full partner in coming to a decision about surgery. "I had a lot of say," she said. "I said 'yes.'" "Suppose you had said no?" "I think my parents and doctors would have sat me down and convinced me, because they really believed that surgery would cure me. This would get rid of the diseased portion of my digestive tract."

Doctors told Sarah she would be normal after the surgeries. They assured her she would be able to do everything her friends were doing. There would be no worries. "I was very excited about that and looking forward to a life with no medicine." Surgery was the end game. "I felt certain the operation would cure me."

Putting away the poison was Sarah's real objective. "I knew I would never have to take those steroids again. Never. That was my motivation." The drugs had taken such a toll on her for so long. "I had come to hate all the drugs." If Sarah made that point once, she did so a hundred times.

The price tag seemed small. "The doctor did not use the word 'downside,' but he said that what you pay is that you go to the bathroom a lot, you get diarrhea a lot." Sarah said she figured that would not be so different from the way she already lived. "I was used to having diarrhea, so that wouldn't have been a huge new thing to deal with. And the drugs would be gone."

Sarah underwent the surgery. Miraculously, her surgeon was able to spare her the ostomy, which meant no bag. "I could not draw you a diagram of what he did, but he avoided a lot of typical things that are done in that kind of surgery."

A day later, a crisis. Doctors detected a problem. They thought there was a leak at the site of the surgery. Maybe this was an opening that had not been properly closed or, because of inflammation, a new hole had opened. "I was rushed into surgery at midnight. They had to call the surgeon, who was home in bed, and he had to race down to the clinic and open me up. Luckily, there was not a leak."

But there was devastating news. A mistake had been made. Sarah never did have ulcerative colitis. The young woman was suffering from Crohn's disease, a similar ailment. The doctors had realized the misdiagnosis only when they reopened her belly. "They said that the Crohn's was evident in the pathology." Sarah was cured of nothing.

Sarah has her own theory. "I think they saw the disease with their own eyes, there in the small intestine." That would be the giveaway. Colitis is limited to the colon, the large intestine. Any sign of disease in the upper GI tract means it is Crohn's.

The prednisone regimen for all those years would have remained because both diseases are types of IBD, and this steroid is standard treatment. The surgery might have been different, although Sarah believes operations would have been in her future anyway. "The mistake was a slap in the face because my expectations were crushed," she says.

Sarah was curiously calm about the misdiagnosis. "This is a very hard diagnosis to make in small children," she explained to me, "and I do not blame anybody. It can take ten years to straighten out." Or longer, in her case.

"Okay, it is a difficult diagnosis in children, but you were sixteen when you went into surgery. You seem to be cutting the doctors a lot of slack for performing what may have been unnecessary surgery."

"I just know it is a common mistake," she said, holding to her line.

"That forgiving, huh?"

"I was angry in general and did not know who to blame." She went on. "This was another case of, why did this happen to me? It never became an issue, like we were going to sue." Finally she admitted to a strong family reaction. "Everyone in our family was angry and very disappointed."

Sarah's father, Paul, weighed in on the subject. "First of all, prior to the surgery, I remember that her colon was nonfunctional. The symptoms were there." Pause. "I have no reason to believe that mistakes were made," the attorney told me. I thought he was pulling his punches.

"Then, why were you angry?"

"This was anger at the situation. Sarah was just devastated when the surgery did not work. We all were."

"Surgery caused more problems than I ever imagined," Sarah said with unusual emotion. "I was sicker than ever. The period after the surgery was the worst, but the bad stuff continued." She battled infections. The dosage of the hated steroids increased.

What once held the promise of a journey's end had become another beginning. Sarah was seventeen and starting her senior year in high school. "Instead of the mind-set that I was going to be better, I had to admit to myself that I was not cured."

Crohn's has a range of severity, with Sarah's case at the wrong end of the spectrum. Her colon, her large intestine, was gone; her small intestine was diseased. "I knew it would get worse and spread to more areas of my digestive tract." How long the promise of no bag would hold is still open to question. "It was a punch in the stomach," Sarah remembered. "I knew there were going to be real hard times ahead."

Interruptions in her life increased. She had been thinking about college and saw more hurdles in her path. "I started missing huge amounts of school and needed tutors." And the terrible side effects of steroids were front and center. "I developed terrible acne again. My face blew up. I had excessive bruising. The mood swings were back, and they were intense." She ticked off her laundry list.

"I was miserable," she said quietly. "The worst depression kicked in."

"You must have been angry," I said.

"My anger comes and goes. As I may have said before,

I hate my body. My body has never done anything good for me."

Dysfunction and discomfort are wearying, compounded daily. Anger and alienation from body, the prison that holds the spirit, imposes a separation from self. I, for one, have painful memories of looking in the mirror after surgery for colon cancer, gazing at the disfiguring bag on my belly. In that moment I felt as the though the real *me* was missing in action. Perhaps my container was somewhere at Baggage Claim, maybe in the hands of aliens. Or terrorists.

"That is how I feel about my body," Sarah wrote in an e-mail one morning. "I am not in control of my body and what it does to me."

"Do you feel alienated?"

"I am detached. You know, I want to trade my body in and get a better, working model."

"Let me know if you find one," I said.

Sarah's view of self had changed. She had always seen herself as different. Now any move toward normalcy was gone. The young woman she has seen in the mirror and rejected over the years was, in fact, her. She was coming face to face with reality. Youth does not accept permanence, never mind the prospect of a compromised life.

Sarah has acknowledged that she sees her life as a one-way trip downward. A remission is possible, she says, but she knows her health will only slide out from under her. "It is inevitable that I will get sick again, and that I will require more surgery," she said with transparent resignation.

"There is no going back." There was a recent three-year gap between hospital incarcerations for her, and she told me she just waits. "I twiddle my thumbs," she sighs, "waiting for things to fall apart again. Not a day goes by for me without thinking about this."

LIFE WOULD GET tougher during Sarah's last year of high school. She was in and out of class, surviving stints at the hospital, relying increasingly on her tutors. "People have said to me, 'Oh, I remember you because you were always sick all the time.' That is sort of what I was known for in those years. That makes me sad that people remember me simply because I was the Sick Girl."

Between relapses, Sarah functioned well. "Every day that I got through without having some sort of crisis or some sort of problem related to my health was a great day," she said, laughing. Between her junior and senior year, she had been well enough to visit Emory University, outside Atlanta, on a college tour.

Sarah struck what her family now calls a victory pose outside a dorm on campus. Arms extended overhead, fists clenched, a broad smile on her face. A photo from that day reveals a determined but frail young woman. That photograph hung on the family refrigerator until Sarah moved into her own apartment, where the snapshot remains on display.

Senior year started well. After intense sickness and tutoring, Sarah had finished the work from her junior year. "All right," she reasoned, "this is going to be a good year. Let's get off on the right foot." But one Saturday morning, she stumbled. She had awakened with the vague sense of just not feeling well.

"I was like, ah, it is sort of my typical morning; I do not

feel good; I will go to the football game and see what happens." A festive atmosphere turned nightmarish for Sarah. Feeling sicker by the minute, she managed to make it home before collapsing. She was rushed by ambulance to a local hospital.

The emergency technicians hollered orders in the screaming ambulance. "You've got to bolus the dopamine faster! Her blood pressure is dropping!" Sarah had gone into shock. "These IVs are not hydrating rapidly enough. I want a central line into her chest now!" That is Sarah's reconstruction of events with her mother's help.

This already fragile young woman had gone septic. Her blood was toxic. The next morning, she was moved by ambulance, again to the Cleveland Clinic. "My blood had been poisoned by a new drug, and I went into multi-organ failure. Everything started shutting down, my kidneys, everything."

She was on the edge. "I am told I was about an hour away from being put on a respirator. The doctor told my parents that I was not going to make it." Then she surprised everyone and rallied. She stayed in intensive care for five days. When she was released and headed home, there was less of her than had left for a football game just days earlier.

"I was so weak that I could not get up the one step from our garage into our house. I remember just sort of crumbling to the ground and crying," Sarah said in a flat voice. "That was when I realized just how sick I had been and how close I had come to not making it."

Sarah did make it. A decade later, the young woman was curled up on her bed on a Sunday afternoon, feeling weak from the regular iron infusion she is given to treat her anemia.

"Did you ever want to give up?"

"No, but I was so scared and drained that I cried a lot, wondering if the rest of my life is going to be like this. I was at my wits' end and did not know what would come next."

"Somehow you muddle through tough situations," I said.

"Yes. I do have to think that."

"And you always will."

"That is how you get through each day." Sarah paused. "Then I meet Crohn's families who have lost kids. It is so sad," she said. "They just go on." Sarah has learned a truth that has kept me going in my struggles with sickness. There is someone out there suffering more than I am.

Sarah suggested that her brush with death became a turning point for a number of her friends. "When these people realized how sick I was, they were shocked. There had been times when we had made plans and I could not go because I did not feel well."

"They did not get it," I guessed.

"Right. They would say, 'Oh, take some Tylenol. You will be fine later.' They did not realize the impact of my illness until they realized that I had almost died." Then they became more compassionate.

Sarah's fixation on the opinions of others continues. "I feel most at ease, I guess, with my old friends," she said. "The newer ones have not seen how sick I can get." She laughed.

"The rest of the world is the problem," I said.

Sarah picked up speed. "Let them feel what it is like to desperately need a nap by two every day. They can swallow sixty pills a day or be on those steroids. Let them see what that does to your psyche."

Self-absorption is emblematic of chronic illness. We become hyperaware of our long siege. Sometimes that is all we can see. And although we will not admit this, sometimes we do feel sorry for ourselves. That others have their own problems and take a less interested view of ours becomes unacceptable. It goes with the territory. Sarah is determined to suck it up and put her best foot forward. As with so many of us who struggle with chronic illness, Sarah badly wants to say the right things and project a calm resolve. Yet knowing that the strong face she shows the world is only a dream suggests how alone she can feel.

SARAH WAS AILING and apart from others during her senior year, staggering but staying on her feet. She was applying to college, badly needing to break away and fly. She occasionally found herself in the hospital that year, battling GI bleeds that would not end. "It was yet another low point," she readily admitted.

"I was in the hospital when I was accepted at Emory. As a matter of fact, I was just out of intensive care. My dad brought me the letter." Sarah had been accepted early decision. She smiled. "I almost had to laugh at how my life was going. That was the only way I could deal with it."

The rest of the year went well. This was the end of an era, she hoped, time to turn the page. "High school was not so much about the lack of freedom. It was just not being able to do things because I was too sick to do them. By the time I went away to school, I was determined to have that normal college experience because my high school experience had been so unusual. I was ready to just fit in and not be the Sick Girl, and just do what everybody else was doing."

Sarah craved and needed a real life existence. She wanted to be part of the social free-for-all most adolescents seek out. For a while, she achieved that dream, acting out like everyone else.

"College is when you are supposed to do stupid things." She giggled. "There were more than a couple of times when I did some stupid things that I should not have done when I was not feeling well. I drank a lot and stayed up until all hours of the night. A lot of the time when I was tired or did not feel well, I just said, 'Screw it. My friends are going out; I am going out with them.'"

The young woman discovered what she was looking for. "Sort of," she laughed, "and there were certainly times when I did not feel happy with myself for the choices I was making." So, take a number and get in line. "But they were my choices, not my mother's."

Sarah was turning into your everyday, stumbling, bumbling college student who just might survive the experience. "For the first time I had periods of time where I was like, wow, I am normal. I am doing what everybody else around here is doing. And I started to feel better about myself."

Sarah was growing, she believes, in an odd way. "I think I went through my developmental stages out of order. When I was fifteen or sixteen, I was sick and was forced to grow up, to be more adult about things. I never had the chance to be the rebellious teenager and do goofy things."

During the last years of high school, illness had kept her on the straight and narrow, even as her parents cut her some slack. They had felt so bad for her that discipline was tough to sustain. "I lied to my parents twice and got caught each time. A few months later I was in the hospital, so that was the end of that."

Atlanta was not totally a crisis-free zone for Sarah. In 1999, when she was a junior, she was in a car accident and sustained a pelvic fracture from her seat belt. "Steroids had softened my bones," she explained. "It is not clear that my pelvis would have fractured otherwise." But aside from the accident, Sarah's college years were relatively uneventful, at least by Sarah standards. "I was in the hospital once or twice a semester," she remembered. "There were the GI bleeds and whatever."

She returned to Cleveland after graduation and enrolled at Case University for a master's degree in social work. During her final semester, the bad combination of a hard Cleveland winter and soft bones led to a fall on some ice. She broke her back and was forced to remain on bed rest for two months, but got herself to commencement.

THEN SHE WAS told by a specialist that she suffered from anorexia. Another brick had been added to her load. The eating disorder is the only piece of Sarah's tarnished health that elicits a self-conscious response. She resists the labeling.

"I will not say I suffered from classic anorexia. My weight did drop to under eighty pounds. My point is that the problem was triggered by events," she explained unconvincingly. "These were mostly breakups with boyfriends, once at the end of college and once again in graduate school."

Sarah concedes that weighing seventy-nine pounds with her already small frame did point to a problem. "Yes, of course it was a problem. I did not want to eat." She insists she was not starving herself. "Some days I ate a little fruit," she argued, "but I never had days when I was eating nothing." If not starving, then what? "I was so depressed. My life was changing before my eyes, and I could not function."

Even as she got over crises in romance, her weight loss continued. She casually mentioned to me that her psychiatrist was the director of the best eating disorder clinic in Cleveland and that he strongly recommended treatment for anorexia. "I was very stubborn."

"You mean you were in denial."

Sarah giggled. "I think I was in denial."

Those around her saw through her refusal to face the music. "They would say, 'Are you kidding me? Look at you.'" Sarah may deny the diagnosis but cannot put aside the problem. She relates her eating patterns directly to the Crohn's. Call it an eating disorder or a really dumb diet, she punished her body because of an image crisis and perhaps because of depression.

"I think subconsciously it is connected to not feeling great on the inside. I do not know that everything is connected, but I think for me it is."

"You mean, to your illness."

"Yeah, the Crohn's has affected how I see my body,

especially with the horrible side effects of those drugs." She is particularly upset about the stunted growth caused by the steroids. "I would be about five feet, five inches tall if I had not been on those steroids."

"That is a big issue for you."

"Yes," she snapped. "People constantly tell me I look like I am fourteen, which makes me really, really angry."

We were driving around Shaker Heights. Sarah elaborated as we headed down the street where she grew up. "I have always looked young. I look at myself," she continued, "and I am not happy. I feel I do not get the respect I deserve."

"Everything just seems to be connected."

"Yeah. I look at myself and I look at my friends, and I do not necessarily think I look younger than my friends, but the rest of the world does. People see me with my friends and think that I am someone's little sister."

"Tell me, why do you measure everything against other people instead of what you yourself want to be?"

There was a silence. "I think probably this is a bit too much about other people," Sarah admitted. "It is stupid that I do that because I compare myself to other people my age who do not have chronic illnesses."

"So, why do you do that?"

"I think I do it without thinking, Oh, I have a chronic illness. That is why." Sarah is surrounded by healthy peers. "I probably mythologize their lives and do not think carefully enough why I cannot have the same." Not only do other young women not enjoy lives as perfect as Sarah imagines but, by any measure, Sarah's life is productive and, by many standards, normal.

"Yeah. I go back and forth in thinking that. It depends what mind-set I am in." Sarah seems to wander all over the map on this. "At times I am okay and do think I am relatively normal," she says without emotion. "I was able to go away to school and travel." She sighs deeply. "On the other extreme, there are times when I feel abnormal and totally different from my friends and other people my age."

MANY OF SARAH'S friends chose to leave home after college, but Sarah returned to Cleveland. "I did have the fantasy, like, wow, I wish I could do that." She giggled. "I still have that fantasy."

Independence at Sarah's age becomes its own endgame. This rite of passage is how young men and women prove to themselves that they are grown up. To stay in the shadow of her parents is to admit she is different. Nevertheless, putting distance between herself and the security of a home that has sustained her is untenable and unthinkable.

"I THINK IT was a fear of finding new doctors," Sarah said without embarrassment. "My mother also would be devastated if I left. She would take it personally."

"Did you stay for her?"

Pause. "It was more for me." Sarah stopped momentarily. "And there was making my mom happy, of course."

Family dynamics in Sarah's home seem frozen in time. Sarah's tie to Mom is center stage, with Dad playing a supporting role. Brother Marshal has disengaged and is gone.

Sarah and I were drinking coffee again at Shaker Square, a few miles from her parents' home. She was preparing me for our pilgrimage to Mom. My trip west had been built around spending time watching mother and daughter interact. After our coffee, Sarah and I headed for Joan and Paul's middle-class homestead in Shaker Heights.

Joan and Sarah sat in the well-furnished family room wrapping small presents for a wedding shower Sarah was planning for a close friend the next day. Shaker Heights is a prosperous tree-lined suburb east of Cleveland, laid out in a uniform grid on land once owned by the North Union Community of the United Society of Believers, known as Shakers, so-named for their shaking bodies during religious dances.

This morning, Sarah sat on the floor, literally at her mother's feet, looking up dutifully. For a self-possessed professional who walks up and down the tough streets of Cleveland, winning the respect of her colleagues, her little girl's demeanor and voice seemed unfamiliar as she asked for guidance about each small detail. Which fancy paper would be used? How should the bows be tied? Sarah was waiting for instructions.

"My mom and I have an interesting relationship," Sarah observed. "Some might say we are co-dependent, even enmeshed." Obviously, this was not the first time these two were discussing this topic. Both women spoke with ease as we discussed how insidiously a chronic illness works its way in to define important relationships.

"In some part, this is the result of my Crohn's and the fact that for a significant part of my life, I only had my parents to rely on."

Joan believes that her aggressive approach has worked for Sarah. "My exacting standards and high expectations have helped Sarah rise to the occasion."

In recent years, Sarah has struggled to break old patterns, if not burst free. "Once I hit my early and mid-twenties, I wanted to make decisions for myself," she said in the family room. Of course, that is what anyone at that age wants. "But by that time, my mom was so involved in my life." Sarah paused, glancing at her mother. "She is a control freak," she added evenly and with no hint of humor as her mom listened without objection. "In the best sense of the word," Sarah threw in, giggling. "It is impossible for my mom to let go and not put her two cents in. Always. 'Oh, you made a mistake.' 'You should have done this or not done that.'" Yet, there was no discernible tension in the room. They had been over this ground before.

But Sarah's baseline of dissatisfaction with the relationship runs deep. "She will constantly say that something I do is immature, something I have said or the way I respond to something is not appropriate or good enough," Sarah continued.

Sarah admitted the criticism can be on target. "Oftentimes it is, but I think it is because even now, at twenty-seven, I am still learning how to be more independent, learning how to say no to my mom." Pause. "No, Mom," Sarah said, turning toward her mother. "This is my life."

For Sarah, this is serious stuff. Steroids cause easy bleeding and bruises. She may want her freedom, but the line between needing help and feeling overly controlled is blurry, particularly when the fight for freedom can come at a steep price. "It has definitely caused a lot of tension in our relationship."

Sarah clearly wants to rewire the relationship. "Most women have mother-daughter relationships that evolve into a friend relationship. I think my mom and I became friends too early, out of need. Then my mom wanted to go back and still mother me and guide me more than I want."

There are no villains here. These are two loving and vulnerable women who cannot seem to break old habits that no longer satisfy. "I need my independence," Sarah said to her mother.

For Sarah, her twenties have been a struggle for separation from a mother who unwittingly may have evolved into being overbearing. "I have this complex dynamic with my mom that no matter what I do, I am never going to be good enough." By now, I was watching Mom. Joan's wince was slight, but she took the emotional fire.

"Sometimes I feel like I am being put down. I feel like I am a failure to her," Sarah finished, turning back to me.

Joan seemed to recognize Sarah's feelings. "The downside of my pushing," Joan said, "might be that Sarah worries about how others will see her if she cannot live up to those high expectations in the future."

A bit self-serving, it seemed to me. Sarah is a grownup, though she does keep going back for more. "I think that is very true," Sarah readily acknowledged. "As much as I, both of us, talk about changing our relationship, we always go back to our same old ways. For the most part it seems to work."

When Sarah and I talked later, I asked if there would be any resolution. Sarah chuckled. "We recognize our patterns and acknowledge who we are. You know, we are never going to fix things. Right?" A pause. "By now it is almost a joke."

A week later I asked more seriously. "Are you both, in your own ways, casualties of chronic illness?" Sarah thought overnight and responded by e-mail.

"I see my friends and other people my age living away from their families, being totally independent, not having to worry about insurance, medical bills, and whether or not they forgot to take a pill at the right time. I wanted to be taken care of again. That is probably when my relationship with my mom really began to veer off course."

Sarah goes back and forth about her mother. "My mom has devoted her life to me and my health care needs. I feel indebted to her." Sarah criticizes her mom, and the guilt sets in. "I feel like nothing I can ever do is going to be good enough to repay her for all she has done for me." Then: "I think she is finally realizing that she needs to take a step back." Finally this: "I do not want you to write anything bad about my mom."

Sarah went on candidly about the state of her emotional heath. "I often wonder what I would be like if I did not have Crohn's, and had not been on steroids for my entire life. Would my personality be the same? Would I be more ambitious, more independent?"

The psychological pressures and problems stemming from this disease can match, maybe surpass, the purely physical. "I think that the emotional side effects have been worse," Sarah confirmed. "Mood swings, depression, irritability, short temper, even distraction when on high doses of prednisone."

These battles of the mind scared Sarah into staying close to home. "Yes," she said slowly. "I think that having parents to rely on for the physical stuff has been important."

Then she switched gears. "I look to them for emotional support," she told me. "There are times that we help each other. We feel crappy together." Does it help? "Yeah," she said. "It makes me feel less alone or even less alienated."

Sarah's condo is located just down the road from her folks, and she is anything but disengaged. After intense consultation with Dad and some financial assistance, Sarah purchased a two-bedroom condo in Mayfield Heights, another suburb of Cleveland. This is a grown-up place, with an attached garage, back porch, and all.

"I always feel like I am a few steps behind everyone, racing to keep up," Sarah said as we sat in the new condo. She seemed to feel she was catching up. "In getting the job and now buying the condo, I do feel closer to the others."

But not enough. "Then reality comes back," she said in a tired voice. "How I feel, my lack of energy and all the problems are still there. I am still behind everyone else. That is why I need my mother."

Living in Levin Land is a mixed blessing. No scenario better demonstrates the co-dependence, an arguable downside to proximity that Sarah and Joan have created for themselves, than the night of the big cleanup. "Sarah had been schlepping herself out of bed every day," Joan said. "'When is she going to clean and do everything?' I asked myself." One can guess the rest. Joan got the job done. "I just could not stand that the floors were dirty and clothes were not washed." Yes, but those were not your problems.

"So, Joan," I ventured, "are you planning to ever give Sarah some room and even stay out of her face?"

"Are you kidding?" she laughed. "I am in there with

both feet." I had the uncomfortable feeling she was not kidding. "You cannot change it," Joan added, "much as I have tried. I do say I am not going to do something. Then I do it and get angry with myself. Then, of course, I rationalize why I did it."

Small wonder Sarah cannot shake her unanswerable questions. "If I were healthy, would we be as close as we are?" she wonders out loud. "Will we always be so codependent?" And the conclusion Sarah had resisted or at least withheld until now.

"I think that if I did not have Crohn's that I would have ventured out on my own after college, far from home. I felt the need to come home because it was safe. I was back in my comfort zone." Case closed. Almost. The impact of chronic illness on a family is powerful. When one family member suffers, family dynamics change, apparently for good. Illness is a shared ordeal.

Paul Levin had always spoken openly about his tendency to allow Joan to take the lead in times of crisis. Now he seemed to feel like an outsider in the discussions of mother and daughter. "I was just talking to my dad," Sarah wrote to me. "He said that he sometimes feels he did not take an active enough role in the medical part of everything, but agreed that he was usually the one who provided more constant emotional support." Weeks earlier, Sarah had characterized Paul as her buddy. "We are pals."

Sarah is circumspect. "With regard to the roles that my family members took on as we dealt with my Crohn's," she said, "I think that everyone fell into the role that he or she was meant to play. My mom was the one most in charge, both of my medical care and my life."

Young Ben Cumbo had expressed his share of anger. I live every day with mine. Sarah does not need a human target for hers, though I think she has identified one. She seems angrier at Mom than she will say.

SARAH'S LARGEST CONCERN is her isolation from others. "There are times since I have been out of college that I have separated myself from the rest of the world. I did not have a lot of friends when I first came back to Cleveland."

That was a strategic maneuver. "I felt like it is a lot easier to not have friends and have to explain my life story. Like, 'Okay, nice to meet you, and this is why some Friday nights I might be tired and not want to go out.'" Sarah seemed tired of explaining her fatigue. "It is very overwhelming," she said in a weary voice. "I had done that in college and I had done that in high school. I am tired of filling everyone in."

Instead, she spent a lot of time with her parents. "Only in the past year or so have I made an effort to isolate myself less and to get myself out there and meet people."

Three years ago, in spite of her self-imposed solitude, Sarah discovered a special man, Ben. The two had met on a Jewish Internet dating site. "She asked me out," Ben kidded, gesturing to Sarah. The three of us were sprawled on couches in Sarah's living room. "I did not!" she yelled back.

"My personal ad said, 'Good things come in small packages.'" Sarah was animated. "She posted a good picture," Ben responded, adding, "She gave me her number but I had to ask her out. Let us just say that Sarah did not make it difficult."

Sarah and Ben are an unlikely couple. Ben is an outdoorsman. Sarah just wants a room at The Ritz. Ben works in the auto insurance industry, in a position he says offers no challenges. The man seems bored with work but captivated by Sarah. They became engaged in February 2006, and married in October.

A serious relationship was a long time coming for Sarah. It was her ticket away from solitude, something she badly wanted. "Seeing my friends start to get engaged and actually get married just made me realize what was missing for me," she told me. Marriage makes her feel whole.

"Being married makes me feel more normal, like I am back on the path of doing what my friends are."

"That matters a lot to you."

"Yes," she responded. "Despite the fact of a serious illness, somebody loves me. I do take great comfort in that."

Sarah had always questioned if she was attractive or appealing, and if somebody would want to date or even have anything to do with her. "I felt that I came with a lot of baggage."

Our culture celebrates physical perfection. Women must be flawless. They are certainly not supposed to go near the bathroom, never mind use it. Sarah knew what she was up against.

A young woman can be as vulnerable to those cultural constructs as anyone on the planet, buying into the preposterously idealized view of her gender. "Not this one," Sarah practically shrieked. She guffawed at the very idea that, given her problems, she conceivably could buy into that glossy magazine stereotype. "A woman burps or passes gas in public," she went on. "Oh, my God, I have never seen a woman do this before." Shocking, isn't it? "There is such a double standard."

"That may be," I pointed out, "but you are its victim."

"One of the first things I used to do is make everything clear when I would first meet someone." Crohn's calls for full disclosure. "Yeah," she responded. "I would say, 'I might fart in front of you, and I go to the bathroom a lot. So, if you cannot handle a woman who does those things, I will not see you.'"

"Sounds like risky business," I said. Throwing down the gauntlet may not be the best way to attract members of the opposite sex. Of course it does identify and separate the squeamish efficiently.

"A lot of guys would say, 'Wow. I am glad you are honest about that.'" Then what happened? "Well," Sarah said without hesitation, "if there was some kind of connection, then we continued dating. I have never had a situation when someone just left because of that."

Sarah was smart to open up about her problems in these social situations. Ultimately, it spared all parties discomfort further down the road. "People have said this is not something you need to talk about on your second or third date." Sarah sounded casual enough but sure of herself.

"I think it is one of the most important things to talk about early." She stopped. "I need to know peoples' initial gut reaction to my illness and how they are going to deal with this stuff." She was not done. "And another thing," she said. "Parents can be the problem. The so-called grown-ups can say, 'We do not want you marrying a sick person.' That is unfortunate."

Sarah summed up her situation. "There are just unpleasant things, which are not ladylike. The physical truth is not something that guys want to think about or deal with. It is a very unglamorous thing."

Sarah made clear that this was not some abstract issue. "It was embarrassing at times, being out on a date and having to go to the bathroom, and spending ten minutes in there, and the guy is wondering what is wrong with you. 'Oh, I had a bad attack of diarrhea.'"

Ben took Sarah to a Mexican restaurant on their first date. That was smart. "I was very concerned about our first meeting because I was on prednisone at the time," Sarah recounted, "and I looked completely different from the picture he had seen. I was afraid he was going to see me and say, 'Oh, my God, who are you? What happened to you?' My face was so puffy."

Each seemed to be trying not to get too serious the first time out. Later in the evening, they moved to a bar. Sarah admits to being a little drunk when she broke the news to him.

"She kind of worked it in, like it was this big deal," Ben interjected. "'There is something I have to tell you,' she suddenly said." Ben could not imagine what he was to hear. "The mind goes wild: What? Does she ha eye? Sarah said, 'I have Crohn's Disease.' Th ing to connect it to."

"Did you run for the fire exit?"

"No," Ben replied. "Why run to spell the disease. I did not k 'It will not be a big deal.' I foun half wrong."

As someone who had gone th

sidered when to reveal the news about my MS, I understood how vulnerable Sarah had felt. You want to do the
right thing but it's hard to know exactly what that looks
like. The information we hide automatically becomes dark
to us, something to fear. We then expect the worst from
others.

"The Crohn's has not affected our relationship at all,"
Ben said almost one year before the engagement. Right, I
said to myself. Stick around. "I do not think I have dealt
with that aspect of our relationship yet," he said two sen-
tences later. I rest my case.

Even in a relationship that offers so much promise, serious illness is difficult to process. Couples genuinely believe
that things will be okay. That they will work it out. Meredith and I discussed my MS in our early years together but
we brushed off the unthinkable too easily. Worst-case sce-
narios do not carry the ring of truth. What might happen
differs from the certainty of what will.

"I have no way of knowing things will be fine," Ben
had said. Ben is a thoughtful and cautious guy. He weighed
each question carefully. "At no time has the disease inter-
fered in a real way. So far it is small stuff, tiredness or bad
moods. Nothing severe."

Intimacy was Sarah's worst fear. "Intimate relation-
ips are very stressful," she had offered. "I worry that
thing is going to happen when we are intimate." De-
re omitted. "At this point, Ben and I are comfort-
gh together that if anything does happen, he will
it. It just takes getting used to."

gh stuff, especially for young people poised
line. Who would disagree that a strong

physical attraction is a defining piece of a romantic relationship? Sarah and Ben are already tailoring their expectations by necessity.

"I think we have a less exciting physical relationship than a lot of people our age," Sarah had said. "But it works for us." She walks back and forth between romance and realism. She accepts the reality of her situation but wishes things were otherwise. "The whole subject can stress me out. Sometimes I have a bad stomachache instead of the headache. So it is, 'Not tonight, dear. I have a stomachache.'"

Sarah thought that was pretty funny. She was serious, though, struggling to see her glass as half full. "Ben and I connect, and we enjoy each other's company on so many other levels. This is not an issue at all," she argued convincingly. "Ben gives me my space."

Despite Sarah's upbeat demeanor, it was clear that this was not an easy subject. "It makes me wonder if we are normal compared to our friends." Again, Sarah fell into her pattern. "I feel like it is disappointing to Ben. Then I transfer that to myself. I feel like I am a disappointment."

"I think the physical relationship matters a lot more to men," I said.

"Yeah," Sarah sighed, "and Ben is a guy."

"Do you sense any dissatisfaction?"

"Ben says, 'No, that is not the case.' I still have that thought in my head." Sarah slowed down. "This relates to the whole body thing. Sometimes I feel bloated and ugly."

"Are you self-conscious with Ben?"

"Mostly I have grown out of it, except when I am having a bad body day."

The subtext for our conversation about intimacy and related issues is that Crohn's disease is a moving target. However slowly the condition progresses, it moves in one direction and will get worse. "I suppose I will have to rise up and meet my piece of the challenges," Ben answered carefully. "If her parents will take care of Sarah's physical well-being, I will do the rest."

Sarah seemed as taken aback as I when she learned of Ben's remarks. "It surprises me a little that he says that. I thought he wanted my parents to be less involved," she said. "Ben probably feels relieved that they will be there. He knows what I have been through and knows there are hard times ahead."

"Is he freaked?"

"No. I think he has begun to prepare himself," she answered and paused. "We do not know how he will react. Probably it is a comfort to know that my parents will be involved. That is not to say he will not take an active role and be a wonderful support."

Ben was not the only family member keeping an eye on evolving roles. Joan's antennae were up. "My fear is that Sarah is going to rely on her husband the way that she relies on me."

"So what is wrong with that? I would think you would want that to happen," I said.

"Truthfully, I do not want her husband to be her nurse-maid. I do not want him to pick up where I leave off."

"Are you worried about getting in over your head?" I asked Ben.

"Not yet, but that could be foolish of me. Look," he added, "I do not like to think of Sarah bedridden and in pain." He thought. "I know that could happen. I only have the smallest bit of knowledge."

The subject seemed to make Ben tense. "I could be fooling myself," he continued. He grasped for an analogy. "This is kind of like a war and being in the trenches. The soldier does not know what is over the hill."

Ben revealed no doubts about his commitment. "None," he said firmly. "I have removed illness from my mind. I set the Crohn's aside and try not to factor it in." That is a dangerous strategy, I silently said. It was time to leave this guy alone. "One more thing," he offered. "We are incredibly communicative. We do a good job of talking."

Ben was learning this: that which is Sarah's will become his. "When you joined my life," Sarah said to Ben. "You acquired a chronic illness. My family already has that chronic illness. It affects each one of us differently, but that is what happens. You have to work it into your relationship and your way of life."

Sarah was determined that this relationship work. She had taken the lead in making Ben comfortable with Crohn's. "Do you feel prepared to deal with the uncertainties of the future and my health?" she asked Ben. "Like the fact that I may have to have more surgery? Have an ostomy?" Ben answered quickly. "Yes. That is something we discussed five months ago." His body language said, "Back off."

Sarah long believed that having children should come before radical surgery, that an ostomy and bag can stifle a sexual relationship. "For me, the fear of an ostomy before I have kids is both psychological and physical. Yes, an ostomy could have an effect on sex."

More finite concerns were in the front of Sarah's mind. "Crohn's can complicate a pregnancy. That is an unknown but a chance worth taking." It comes down to the strength of the desire for children. "Ben and I want kids, and it is possible we can pull it off before there is any more surgery."

The clock is ticking. "We want to have children in the next couple of years. I think I maybe can hold off an ostomy for that long." That would be pretty cool. "That would be very cool." The focus, rightfully, was on Sarah. Ben's role as partner and source of support carries its own complications.

Five years from now, and perhaps forever, questions will remain. What any of us believes about taking on a spouse who is suffering from a serious illness is continually tested. We all want to be partners and lovers, not caseworkers. Our notions of what is rewarding and important will determine if the sacrifices we make are worth it.

Sarah and Ben took me to California Pizza, jammed with young people obviously hipper than I. It was a struggle just to walk in, never mind stand around and wait for a table. I could not move, but that was okay. I could not hear, either. I watched Sarah and Ben. There was an ease about them.

"I am in awe every day that you stay with me," Sarah told Ben. "I feel that I come with so much baggage, that I am a defective person. It amazes me that you are still around." Sarah's words had that sense of astonishment, as if she and Ben lived in a dream from which she expected to awaken.

That insecurity rings true. "There is always a part of me that is waiting for the bubble to burst," she said in a matter-of-fact voice. "Sometimes I think there are too many good things in my life." That last sentiment contradicted many that had come before.

"And you have been burned before, right?"

"Yes."

Sarah's illness had barged into relationships before. "This is different. I have never been more secure. I know Ben is not going anywhere." That calm confidence, too, seemed out of character.

On our long ride back to my hotel that evening through Shaker Heights, I asked Ben if illness had made Sarah insecure. Ben responded instantly. "If I saw Sarah through her own eyes, I do not think I would want to be with her."

"But . . ." I said, leaning forward to coax the thought.

"But I see her through my eyes, and I am trying to get her to see herself that way." Then Ben turned slightly toward Sarah, in the backseat. "I want to work my magic and make you see yourself in a new light." He laughed softly. "I think this is going to take a while."

He pulled the car into my motel's parking area, and we kept talking for a few minutes. "Sarah is a good person," he said. "Thank you," she said back. Ben laughed. "And she knows what she wants and goes with her gut. I do not," he chuckled. "She dives into the pool. I am testing it with my toe." Ben was not hanging around just to play nursemaid. The young man got something he needed from Sarah.

Ben expressed a last, unsolicited sentiment before driving off into the darkness. "When Sarah is happy, I am happy," he said. "When Sarah is grumpy, I find alternative ways to bide my time." Ben laughed. Sarah betrayed a faint smile. She knew what he meant.

"Is a sense of humor important to you guys?" I asked.

"Capital Y, Yes, for sure," Ben responded, though he implied that his jokes can fall on deaf ears. "Sadly, I am my best audience." Then they each laughed. "Sarah cracks me up, too, which is nice. This has nothing to do with her Crohn's. Sarah is a klutz."

Sarah giggled. "If we did not laugh," she added, "we would be crying a lot."

EVEN THOUGH SARAH is frequently upbeat, clinical depression has opened another front in what has become a very long war in such a young life. Her depression is not just related to her Crohn's. Clinical depression runs in Sarah's family, primarily on her mother's side. But the role of Crohn's in the mix has to be a strong factor. Sarah believes that Crohn's, in fact, triggers a genetic predisposition for depression.

"Did my illness trigger my depression gene? Did it stem from the steroids, or was it situational depression? I think it is a question that I will ponder for the rest of my life and take with me to my grave, which I do not plan on visiting for a very long time."

What kinds of events provoke the depression? "Little things do, like coming home from work any day of the week, maybe with plans, and being so exhausted that I just have to get into bed and cannot fathom doing anything that night. That is when I'm like, ech, what is wrong with me?"

"You sound just plain weary."

Sarah offered her take. "It does sort of feel like there has been a black cloud over me for pretty much all my life. As soon as one thing is fixed, the next thing breaks. As soon as I am back on my feet from one episode, I get in my car accident or I fall and break my back." Chronic illness, we learn the hard way, knows no end. "My friends know but do not get it and just do their thing."

"I knew after the surgery that I was a few degrees off-center." Meaning? "Looking back, I think it was not so clear, but I was not feeling right." Illness-related issues may have touched off the explosion, but the depression was there. "I think if there were no disease, I would have had bouts of mild depression." We will never know.

Those who suffer from severe chronic illnesses can fall victim to secondary crises that follow not far behind. Signals can be subtle, problems slow to spot. "Things that once made me happy did nothing for me anymore." Such as? "My brother and I were looking at cars. My parents were going to buy one for us to share at the end of high school." Sarah remembered that a happy process became joyless.

"We were looking at Pathfinders. I loved that particular car. It just did nothing for me anymore. Something was wrong. I was numb. I started seeing a social worker, who I did not like too much. The whole thing was too touchy-feely for me, so I moved to a psychiatrist." The doctor thought Sarah's psychological problems were at least partially situational, Sarah's term for Crohn's-related depression.

"I started taking medication. Antidepressants." Sarah's psychiatrist had confirmed the depression diagnosis.

Sarah's physical health had been pretty good for a while. "Yeah, but I had those bouts with not eating and became an emotional mess."

Many of us who deal with chronic illness are dealing with a cumulative burden, greater than the sum of its parts. It stands to reason if you put enough weight on your back, sooner or later it can be hard to stand up. "Just thinking back on everything that I have been through makes me depressed," says Sarah. "The whole 'woe is me' reaction is not my thing, but there are days when I want to say that."

"There have to be days when people like us say 'poor me' in our heads, if not aloud."

"Exactly," Sarah echoed. "I break down to my parents, but . . ."

"That does not count," I interjected.

"Right," Sarah responded quickly. "But with my friends and stuff, I would never say it."

"Why?" I wondered. "These are your friends, your support system."

"I try to put on a brave front," Sarah answered. "I do not want them to think I am a complainer." She has been there for them. "Yeah, and it is frustrating because I lend a shoulder for others to cry on when things are bad." She paused. "No one understands anyway, so what is the point?"

Sarah continued. "I guess my Crohn's constantly makes me second-guess myself and question who I am. It is a very unsettling feeling to constantly wonder who I am and might be if my situation were different." That, of course, is a fruitless inquiry.

"I am very scared for what is going to come next and when it is going to show up and what it is going to be." Those who suffer serious sickness know there is an ambulance with their name on it, parked just around the corner. "I imagine further surgeries and further complications. Cancer, probably. I am more likely to get some sort of GI-type cancer than the average person. Statistics show that." Cancer festers in Sarah's head, but she is too smart and strong to go there for long.

The lady continues to be tougher than she appreciates. A single-minded drive for success has carried her through operating rooms and into the schoolrooms of her chosen work. Her selection of a career path suggests a concern for others, even as she is absorbed by her own trials. Sarah's stealth steeliness has served her well.

We visited the Beech Brook agency near Shaker Square in Cleveland. The renovated building houses school-based programs and out-patient services. I watched Sarah mingling with colleagues, filing reports, calling clients. The lady was all business.

"It is hard to know how Sarah keeps going," I said to her former supervisor.

"It is this incredible desire to be like everybody else," the woman responded, smiling. "Nothing is going to stop her, no matter what it is." Even physical relapses. "Sarah has this drive," she continued. "She says, 'I know it is bad, but I am not going to let it get me.'" Sarah's old boss laughed softly. "Sarah is like the Energizer bunny."

"Do you think illness has made Sarah a better person?"

"Illness probably made her more mature than a lot of people her age. Part of this may be a result of what she has been through." She does seem determined. "Sarah seems undaunted by what life has given her."

"I will bet she is better with clients for her own struggles."

"Sarah has an empathic nature that I believe has been supplemented by her own struggle."

What motivates Sarah, her friends believe, is that strong desire to be like everyone else. One might call that healthy. Sarah's lifelong obsession with being known as the Sick Girl misses the point. Sarah is the sick girl who is building a healthy life.

One major skirmish remains, what may be the final battle of a long war. The prospect of that last surgery weighs heavily on her. The operation will change her life, probably for better and worse.

"I think it is inevitable that I will end up with an ostomy. I really do."

An ostomy. The prospect must be horrifying. Human waste goes out the front of the belly and directly into a bag. Those of us who have undergone the procedure, even temporarily, know all too well that we are not talking about just a bag. This is *The Bag*.

Sarah has no colon, so she cannot have a colostomy. Hers, if and when it comes, will be an ileostomy, the fast-track from small intestine to bag. That means waste leaves the body earlier in the digestive process. "My whole rectum is so diseased," Sarah said simply.

"I am realizing that we have been trying to put Band-Aids on, and it is not working. The doctor has told me the next surgery I will have *is* the ileostomy. It is going to happen, whenever." That sounds like a done deal. "No,"

Sarah answered quickly, as if she wanted to shout, "Don't say that." "No," she repeated. "God willing, there will be progress, or they may find a cure."

The young woman paused. "The disease will continue, and I will get worse. I know that. I go through cycles of thinking. I see crazy mental pictures of what it will be like."

"You still hold out hope." "Not really. Well, yes I do. I do not know."

As a cancer survivor and alumnus of the temporary ostomy class of 2000, I cannot imagine dealing with the permanent procedure. "I cannot even wrap my head around that right now," Sarah added. "It is very scary." The question is what a bag will do, psychologically. "Nothing good," Sarah said. "I think because I am married, it will be much easier. But in terms of my body issues, I cannot imagine what it will do."

The bag will create a new awkwardness. "I am uncomfortable enough with my body already," she noted. "To think about life like that, about being intimate, is very hard. I do not know how I will ever get used to the whole thing." Turn your imagination loose. "I picture this big bag of poop that I am carrying around, just hanging off of me."

Sarah suddenly laughed out loud, as if the idea seemed nothing less than preposterous. "I think that what is in my mind is worse than it would be," she admitted. "A bag can be discreet. It comes in different sizes and you even can wear a bathing suit. But I would rather continue bleeding and feel like crap, at least at this point, than go down that road."

"A lot of people have gone through this," I told Sarah.

"I guess I will have to," she responded with a deep sigh. "I know people who have had this for over twenty years now. Some have adjusted pretty well." She stopped. "Actually, two of them still have bad problems. Others seem to have totally normal lives." In Sarah's mind, the jury is still out.

"Ben will be involved in the decision," she continued. "He knows it probably is inevitable. Ben says whatever needs to be done to make me feel healthy and well, he supports, whatever the decision." This was sounding too easy.

Sarah agreed and wanted to get into the details with Ben. "I was trying to make the point that if and when this surgery happens," Sarah wrote, "it is not going to be like someone snapped his fingers, and all of the sudden my quality of life is improved one hundred percent, and everyone is happy and goes on their merry way."

She went on. "I explained that recovery from a GI surgery is long, painful, frustrating and, more than anything, disgusting. I was not sure he was getting what I was trying to say, that it was going to take a looooonnnnggg time to get there. Finally, he basically said 'Do you think I am stupid?'"

Sarah needed to push harder. "'What if, during the night, my ostomy bag breaks, or I have some sort of accident? Do you understand that this is going to happen from a surgery like that?' His response (no joke or pun intended) was, 'I do not give a shit. IT IS JUST SHIT. We will clean it up and move on.'"

Wow.

On the last day of my final visit to see Sarah, the two of us drove to the Cleveland Clinic, where Sarah has been treated for more than a decade. The Clinic is an imposing complex on the city's east side. We headed for the Pyramid Building, a pointed glass tower encased in a web of steel. The lobby was teeming with people moving in and out, heading for elevators on their own steam, or with canes or crutches, or in wheelchairs.

Sarah was headed to her gastroenterologist for a regular checkup and took me along. The doctor, a Mexican Jew of Eastern European descent, had a gentle way with Sarah, and her trust in him was clear. The doctor knew she and I had been discussing the dreaded ileostomy.

The man did a quick exam, then began working on Sarah gently, making a case for the surgery. No time frame was discussed. There was no pressure. The doctor knew it would take courage for Sarah to go through with the operation, whenever the time did arrive.

"I believe that people develop a strength that is related to quality-of-life issues," he said to Sarah as he sat before a computer. "That is easy for me to say, I know, because I am sitting on the other side of that issue." The tone seemed almost casual. His accent was pronounced, his voice, soothing.

Sarah was focused on the doctor's every word, as if straining to be convinced. He told her there was one method for approaching the surgery for those who feel unsure, almost a halfway measure. "Sometimes doctors try a temporary ostomy, just to see how the patient copes with it," he said. "There are patients who just will not accept having a stoma," the piece of intestine that pops through the belly, to which the bag is fastened.

Before the surgery, the doctor said evenly, "Many Crohn's patients become prisoners in their houses. They have to go to the bathroom every fifteen or twenty minutes, even if it is to pass small spurts of mucus or blood.

"Crohn's is not a deadly disease," he went on. "People do not die from it." Complications of Crohn's can kill, however. Sarah has seen that in her world. And the illness does alter lives. "Once these patients have an ostomy, they can go and have dinner and go to the movies. Their life expands and improves." There was resignation hanging in the room.

"I think the surgery will improve the quality of my life," Sarah offered without conviction on the elevator down. "But will it be worth it? I do not know." She shrugged. "What if there is just more disease and there are more problems?" She shrugged again.

We ambled across the lobby. Sarah continued to seem subdued. "We can get rid of the diseased rectum," she said. "I know that. The Crohn's is just going to crop up somewhere else in my body. I know that, too." I felt bad. The young woman seemed quietly distressed. "What is the point?" she asked rhetorically. "How many more surgeries are there going to be down the line?"

SARAH'S DAD AND I hoofed it up Pennsylvania Avenue, ascending Capitol Hill behind Sarah and the others on a hot, early-summer day months later. We were going to meet with Senate staffers to discuss research on inflammatory bowel diseases (IBD). Folks from around the country had traveled to Washington, D.C., to lobby for more research money. We had split up by state after breakfast and a briefing to head off and plead for support.

"Are you here lobbying for MS?" a woman in line for coffee at a Senate cafeteria asked me. "No, for Crohn's and colitis," I answered, adding, "We all have to stick together." She appeared confused, but nodded. Senate staffers are used to legions of lobbying amateurs trooping through to ask for assistance in fighting every known disease.

Ohio's delegation included a mother who had lost a son to Crohn's only months before these meetings. This dignified middle-aged woman was controlled as we met with aides to her senators, but the tears came as she discussed the tragedy in her family and the human toll of IBD. Her college-aged son had died in a hospital bed, fighting an infection that could not be stopped. Sarah had come close to such a death more than once.

As Sarah and I walked together down long corridors connecting offices in various buildings, we talked about hope. I now understood why she was trudging around Washington. For years Sarah has been an effective advocate, speaking out in Cleveland and elsewhere, winning recognition and awards. Most of all, though, she has touched and been touched by real people.

Sarah said, "Parents of younger children come up to me crying and saying, 'This disease has been so hard on our child, but it is so comforting to know you have been through all of this, and you are where you are today.'"

Sarah shared another observation she hears, no doubt a source of satisfaction. "'You are living your life, succeeding at being as normal as possible.'"

Normal. The magic word. "Beyond normalcy, Sarah, what are your hopes?"

"It is weird," she said. "Sometimes I do hold onto hope, sometimes, I just do not." As with many of us who suffer, Sarah knows that hope is more for future sufferers, not just for us. "You know, for me, things have gone way past any hope for a cure."

We offer lip service to the hope for a cure. Resolution may be around the corner, we assure each other and even tell ourselves. But we do not really think help is on the way.

"My life is what it is," Sarah said a bit bleakly. I know that feeling. MS may be cured, but not in time for me.

"I do have the hope that others do not have to live with Crohn's. My hope for others is stronger than any hope for me."

"What about your kids? There has to be hope on that front."

Sarah was silent. Then, "I hope all kids can have more treatment options and a cure in their lifetimes. I do have major fears that I will give birth to kids who carry that gene." Earlier generations of the Levin family have dealt with Crohn's. "I do not think I would ever get over the guilt."

The delegation broke for lunch. The Levins and I walked one last corridor and parted company. Sarah and her dad headed across Capitol Hill to the House side to grab lunch and gently twist a few more arms. I walked into the heat, crossing a park to head into Union Station and find a train to New York.

I was wearing the electric-purple advocacy bracelet Sarah had placed on my wrist before heading to the Hill. The wristband reads, quite simply, GOT GUTS.

....

Reflections

Living with Grace

Sarah's story teaches that we sick must make peace with our bodies, no matter how uneasy and regardless of how they torment us. Sarah hates the body in which she must live. That container has betrayed her for a lifetime, offering little but physical and emotional pain. Instead of quietly simmering, Sarah expresses elegant contempt for the damaged body in which she is locked.

The toll for Sarah has been heavy because subtle disfigurement, weight gain, and even slightly distorted facial features are not acceptable for women in a culture of narcissism. In a world with such narrow standards of beauty, those who so clearly do not conform are seen as untouchable.

Sarah is young, yet she controls anger with more equanimity than this middle-aged man can muster. High emotion does not get the best of her, yet her feelings are undeniably strong. How she negotiates the wake of disappointment as she plows ahead speaks volumes about living with grace and beauty from within.

Sarah was the first patient selected for this book. I had lived my own edition of her story and known embarrassment and shame. I needed to know how another gets by. With Sarah, I was part voyeur, part student. I watched as she saw her body through the eyes of others. She does not let go of the comparison contest she cannot win. Yet somehow she is able to rise above the hurt.

Her perspective comes from understanding the world around her. As a social worker, she knows that poverty and illness have much in common and that so many of us live in pain. There is no hierarchy of suffering, no sense that anyone's journey is harder than another's. In the end, there is only one life, and hurt will not stop Sarah from living it well.

six

Larry Fricks

Surviving Stigma

LARRY FRICKS AND I drove into a remote southern town to arrive at what was once Georgia's most notorious mental institution, Central State Hospital. The institution dated back to the early 1800s, and once carried the quaint name Georgia Lunatic Asylum. That day, the mammoth buildings of the old institution stood silent, as if they belonged in mothballs.

At one position near a long incline, a 360°-degree pan revealed endless fields of graves extending in every direction. Nothing about any of the simple graves said anything of their occupants. Religious symbols were conspicuously absent. "The graves were not worthy of being protected and kept up," Larry Fricks explained. "Many markers were pulled so they could mow the grass. Even in death, these folks were just forgotten."

The man tried to hold back tears. "Growing up," he

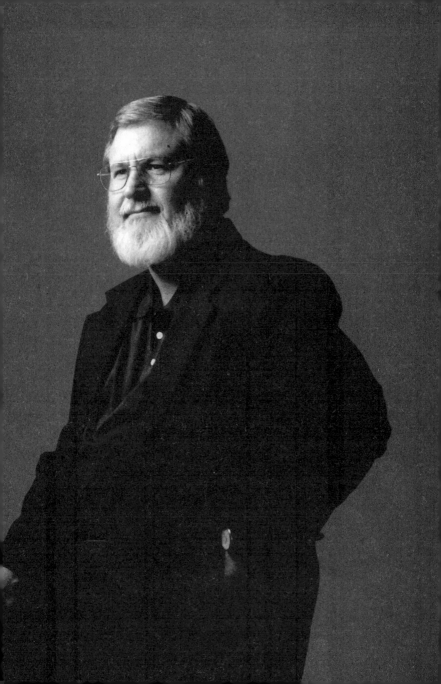

began again calmly, regaining composure, "I was taught that out of respect, not to even step on graves. It is acknowledgment that a human has lived on this earth and that we are all connected."

Over the years, the hospital became known simply as Milledgeville, after the town where it is located. "Behave yourself, children," the admonition went, "or you are going to Milledgeville." Generations of Georgians still talk about hearing that threat and calling a halt to their bickering.

The place was quiet and deserted on this silent September Sunday but still it was imposing, even threatening. The drab stone structures had been home, or rather prison, to almost fifteen thousand troubled souls at any given time. The hospital had been a warehouse for the mentally ill.

Milledgeville became a freak show in Georgia culture. Tourists flocked to the grounds to take in the sights. The facility housed the largest kitchen in the world, an awesome attraction on the school trip circuit. Larry's voice choked as he spoke of the hospital's horrible history.

Electroshock therapy, routinely administered with portable units transported around the floors, was a prime means of maintaining order. One amused superintendent is said to have routinely lavished praise on the "Georgia power cocktail." Psychiatrists were heard, infamously, to demand of patients, "Did Georgia Power make a Christian out of you today?"

Larry brought me there because the history and meaning of the spot have haunted him for decades. "This place is the story of stigma," he explained. "People were brought here and told that they have no role on earth anymore." He paused. "This could have been my home if I were not white and middle-class and reasonably connected." He paused again. "I am mentally ill."

ONE AFTERNOON, MORE than a year earlier, Larry and I had parked among the SUVs and pickups in front of Ma Gooch's Restaurant in Cleveland, Georgia. We sat in the front seat for a while, just down the steep dirt roads from Larry's Appalachian cabin, northeast of Atlanta. We chatted on various subjects, though not about the point of our meeting.

A tentative quality to our new relationship was keeping Larry at a distance. Finally, we ducked into the small joint for a quick lunch. "I eat three meals a day," Larry offered in response to nothing.

"Diet is part of recovery," he went on. I nodded, and stared at him. He looked like a cross between Santa Claus and a lumberjack with his bushy white beard, checkered shirt, and suspenders.

He continued to explain the importance of discipline, ensuring enough sleep as well as establishing a proper diet, in managing a mental illness. "We can do a lot for ourselves." A step-by-step strategy, a commonsense system of maintaining equilibrium and keeping an eye out for any blinking warning signs, is critical. "Vigilance becomes vital," he declared.

Larry was taking it slow, hanging back and feeling me out. To do so seemed second nature for a man accustomed to fending off public ignorance of mental illness. This is a mighty slow dance, I thought as I stared at my unwanted soup. Since my colon cancer, I eat just about nothing during the day. Though soft-spoken and serious, Larry was good company, easy and empathic and warm to the people he encountered. Still, he was guarded with me.

Larry has bipolar disorder, once known as manic depression. He seemed old beyond his fifty-seven years, having traveled to hell and back. A map of his journey is visible in the lines across his face, there to read in his eyes.

Larry had been a young man when the terrible trip began. His dreams were crushed and the bright future that had been his ceased to exist. Mental illness became not an issue in his life but life itself. Even so, his demons are controlled now. He has become a master of self-protection in an unkind world. For him, this acquired skill came the hard way.

When we first met face-to-face in Washington, D.C., a few months before my trip to Georgia, I felt an instant connection. I trusted Larry's drawl, the look in his eyes. We got down to business in his hotel room, words flowing tentatively, a tape recorder humming.

Larry wanted to explain his hesitation to share details of a deeply troubled period in his life. I was frustrated, ready for the flow of information. Conversations with Buzz had been tough. Buzz always stopped at first base, where God seemed to be coaching. Maybe Larry would swing for the fence.

"Please understand, Richard, I am somebody who went to the University of Georgia. I had good jobs and a lot of successes. I made money," Larry said earnestly, getting warmed up. "Even with all that, after I was hospitalized, I was dumbstruck by the sense of hopelessness that people attach to mental illness and the message that came through to me."

The man's resentment at being marginalized was clear.

We agreed to meet again in rural Georgia, Larry's mountainous backyard. Soon enough, Larry's well-worn VW Beetle was climbing into the foothills of the Appalachians toward his cabin on Buzzard Mountain. This was redneck country right out of *Deliverance*. "Scared?" he asked with a smile.

Once we left the highway, the population thinned and the road surface changed to dirt. We passed the trout pond at Turner's Corner, and the incline grew steeper. Larry's house appeared around the last bend through the trees. It was a rustic structure with an addition that looked as if it had been grafted on. A hunchback house.

We got out of the car, and two roaring beasts disguised as dogs walked in circles to check out the Yankee. Losing interest quickly enough, they sprawled around us as we sat on the old wooden porch, sipping lemonade in the warmth of a late-spring afternoon.

Later that night, we drove to the top of his property. We sat again, this time on a craggy hilltop beneath a clear sky. Larry had built an open geodesic dome that towered over us.

"Energy conservation is a piece of my spirituality," he explained. "Doing the right thing in the universe matters." We sat braced against the cold, leaning into a roaring fire as we devoured s'mores.

"So, let's start at the beginning," I said.

"Richard, that is a novel idea," he answered with a smile.

LARRY GRADUATED IN 1972 from the University of Georgia with a major in journalism. By his own account, he was a party animal. "I had grown up Baptist. We did not drink. In college, I discovered alcohol," he said. "There was peer pressure to party, and I joined a fraternity. I even became rush chairman."

In the summer after his sophomore year, he had the first of a series of profound religious experiences. He was working for an electrician in Athens, where the university is located, and was sent to a church to help replace some old wiring.

Larry had time on his hands and nothing on his mind. "I was only a gopher," he explained. He stood around, holding ladders and tools for long periods of time. "I looked, stared, really, at all kinds of stained-glass windows and took in the ambiance." And?

"Something just came over me," he recalled. "I felt an internal awakening, and it was profound at that moment. I had been an acolyte as a Baptist, always wanting to be connected. What happened was not so surprising." Different? "Yes. I felt the presence of God." Buzz would call that the presence of the Holy Spirit. "It felt real."

Might that even have been an early sign of manic behavior? "No," Larry countered, shrugging. "But my older brother certainly now sees this as a sign of things to come." Larry put the moment into the context of the local culture. "This is a rural area and very Christian. This stuff happens to people all the time." He chuckled. "Look. It did not matter, anyway. Months later I was drinking and dancing, you know, partying and back to the old lifestyle." Larry said there may have been other, more classic, signs of manic tendencies back then. He points to his unusual high energy and productivity in college.

"I started a little business back then. I sold party favors and flowers for college events. I just went around and got orders from fraternities and sororities. We did pretty well."

"Can you infer anything from that?"

"Maybe." Larry paused. "I was beginning to speed up. Who knows what it meant?"

If Larry was accelerating, it was not a quick trip from zero to sixty. The move to mental disruption can come slowly.

After graduation, he was heading for another business opportunity when he got drafted and went into the army. "I did the six part-time years, with six months full active duty, and then two weeks in the summer."

Larry had been a child of the sixties, partaking of the indulgences of the time while he was still in school. "I was smoking pot, listening to the Beatles, letting my hair down." Still, there was the vague outline of a plan for the future, and any counterculture habits Larry had acquired would take a backseat to his drive to succeed.

Larry went into the real estate business with Glen, a high school pal. Glen's father was a successful businessman. The possibility of an ice-skating rink somewhere in the Georgia heat took center stage.

"Glen's dad thought it was a great idea." Larry laughs. "It probably was not such a great plan, but, boy, it was a way to meet beautiful women." In fact, Larry had no business experience. But the partners built a rink they called Iceland and did the interior by hand. Then the duo successfully negotiated a deal with the Atlanta Flames, a National Hockey League team, to move hockey practices from another rink to their new facility. Larry did business with the team's trainer. "We gave him a washer and dryer to clean the jerseys. We were rolling," Larry chuckled.

The Atlanta Flames grew into a glamorous and highly visible presence. Amateur hockey at the rink exploded. Larry was night manager and worked his way up to general manager. Finally, he became president of the business.

These were heady days, but psychological disaster was incubating. The presence of the Flames brought a faster life, and Larry began heading for the falls, all the while thinking he was only swimming in the fast lane. His pace quickened, and was easily explained away as strong and positive behavior for a young man in a hurry.

"My energy level was extremely high," he remembered. "I was always on the go. I remember a couple of people shaking their heads and going, 'Man, playing hockey and then going straight to play in a rugby game. Those are pretty strenuous sports.'" He grinned. "They are. But I had an energy level to do it, and I just kept going and going." He was exhilarated. Mania was a mesmerizing, natural high. "It was great," he said. "I felt so good. Man, there was no problem as far as I was concerned."

Larry was a high roller now, going to fancy parties in the moneyed neighborhoods of Buckhead, an upscale section sitting in a northwest pocket of the city. He spent evenings, if not entire nights, barhopping with beautiful women. The high energy of his mania registered with everyone around. "The aura is attractive," Larry said.

All systems were go. But you can only go for so long. Larry began drinking heavily, as an antidote to the high. "When your mind is racing and you have all this intense energy and you need to slow down, to sleep, that is what you do. See, I probably started self-medicating then." I thought self-medicating was only a euphemism for overindulging. "No. I had to come down. Bad."

"The other side of being revved up is that you come down," Larry went on, "but you do not want to move too far down. That becomes depression." Larry began doing drugs to shoot himself back up. "Does this make sense to you, Richard?" I nodded. "This is not a logical dynamic," Larry said.

The formula eventually stopped working. "Alcohol appears to help, but in the end, drinking does not do any good because while it may slow you down and help you fall asleep, ultimately, it is not good for sound sleep," he continued. Many of us learn that on our own. Drinking and awakening in the dead of night become debilitating. "I think the best I was doing was taking the edge off some mania." Self-medication grew into sleep deprivation, which only exacerbated Larry's condition.

The alcohol addiction was compounded by Larry's growing taste for cocaine. "A couple of the ex-Flames I knew would snort it with me." As part of the party scene, Buckhead was a hot spot for cocaine. "You could party all night. I had all the energy I needed." The pull was irresistible. "When you are in the middle of that stuff, that kind of life of privilege, everything centers on lifestyle."

The ice skating rink and surrounding land were sold in 1982. Larry was thirty-two. The sale made financial sense because the real estate was now worth more than the business. Larry shared in the profits from the deal, making two hundred thousand dollars. A short time later, he got married.

Clementine was the wealthy young woman Larry met on the social circuit, wooed and wed. The couple had been on the make, flying high on the Buckhead scene. After the wedding, the pair settled in a wealthy area of town. "We were the entitled. Hell, Richard, we owned two homes in Buckhead."

The couples' friends were the movers and shakers, part of the social elite. "We had been told that someday we were going to have it all." Larry paused. "In fact, we were going to own it all." How did it all feel? "Not all good," he said. "It was a reach for me. My dad was a navy officer. We were middle class."

"But it was also seductive."

"Are you kidding?" Larry laughed. "Hanging out with beautiful people felt good. The rest just melted away."

What no one knew, least of all Larry's partners, was that Larry had embezzled ten thousand dollars from Iceland to underwrite the high life. He had justified the theft, telling himself he was just borrowing the money and would pay it back.

"It did not feel right," he told me, "though my guilt was not about the money but what I had done to my partners." When the rink and surrounding land sold, no one was the wiser. The secret remained locked away in Larry's conscience.

Larry said he had no moral compass and no job. Still, the couple was financially secure. Clementine, whom everyone called Kimi, had a sizable trust fund, and the couple wanted for nothing. In addition to the two Buckhead properties, Kimi and Larry owned a house on Lake Lanier, exclusive property on the Atlanta watershed. The two kept a boat. The partying continued. Yet there was an unsettling feeling hanging over them, a lack of purpose.

Larry joined a favorite uncle in a venture manufacturing women's blouses. From the beginning, the business had big problems and only stumbled along. "I think we had not thought out the concept well enough. Oh boy. I got involved in something that I had no experience in." Larry remembers the enterprise as very stressful.

He and Kimi took a vacation, fleeing to the Fiji Islands in early 1984. For three weeks, the two hiked through paradise. "We were very happy," Larry said. "Kimi even made the comment that it was the happiest she had ever been. We were very much in love." As the couple was touring local exotica, word arrived that Kimi's father had died. "We were stunned but could not get back in time for the funeral," Larry said.

When they did pack up and return, a change in Larry became apparent almost immediately. Paradise was far behind, enormous stress surfaced from the hated blouse business, and his secret about the stolen money and guilt about his excessive lifestyle added to the weight of the load.

An explosion shook their lives.

"I HAD A spontaneous, spiritual awakening, a conversion experience." The power in Larry's voice was unmistakable. "It was like a sustained flash of light. All of a sudden, I broke out in a sweat." Events played out over a three-day period. "I felt that I was wrestling with the deity, and at the end of the third day, I was just certain that God existed," Larry recalled. "God had communicated with me and touched my life, and suddenly, all that mattered was that relationship."

Larry insists to this day that the conversion experience was real, but an intense relationship with the Lord is a classic manic scenario. "It did happen, Richard."

"Or you think it happened."

"This event was the most transformative of my life." Larry is insistent on that truth. "These religious experiences change people," he said quietly. "I still believe that there is a spiritual realm. For me it started with good and evil and the Southern Baptist Church." I just listened. "Apart from my behavior, a lot of things were becoming focused. It was a sense of, oh my God, I have missed a relationship with God in my life, and here it is."

Larry had no strong personal faith at the time, no active religious affiliation that meant anything to him. "We were not active in any kind of church. The conversion seemed to be about God, not about a religion." In reality, of course, the awakening was about Larry.

"God was actively in my life and communicating directly to me," he explained. Our conversation grew intense during a drive through the mountains one sunny afternoon. The great outdoors, the bucolic countryside, could take us seamlessly to the doorstep of God in these talks.

"This was just part of my thought process, asking questions and then providing mental answers. As I got used to it, I was faster at it." Larry was silently reasoning with the Lord. "Richard, that dialogue gave me a superhuman strength. It hooked me into a power I cannot describe. If you believe God is communicating with you, and I did, you feel invulnerable to just about anything."

Larry celebrated the new relationship. "Yes, I did, wholeheartedly. Joyously. This was psychosis, of course. It is not uncommon for people with this kind of illness to have religious conversion experiences and awakening where they think that God is communicating not just with the world but to them directly. But it was real to me."

Larry was convinced that God had a mission for him. He told Kimi that he had been touched by the Lord. Kimi was stunned and frightened for him. The reaction was compounded by her long-standing aversion to Christianity. Kimi stayed silent, though, unsure of how to process Larry's experience.

"But as the behavior became bizarre because of what I believed God was communicating to me, I think it overwhelmed her." There was no time for reassurance. "I went off on my mission to serve God. I was on a roll that lasted for months."

Loose-cannon communications with God were traveling close to the edge. The assumption might have been that Larry had become just another born-again Christian. But Kimi saw nothing routine about the conversion. She was unnerved. And Larry was growing only more intense.

Bubbling over with enthrallment, Larry developed an appreciation for the forgiveness Christ taught and was ready to take care of old business. "I had to seek forgiveness for stealing the money," he said. "I knew that. The time had come."

He set up a meeting to tell his old partners about his misdeed.

"Did you go into that meeting believing God was at your side?"

"I was very frightened," Larry answered, correcting me. "But my relationship with God was the most important factor. Kimi also went to the meeting."

"Who else was there?"

"The stockholders were all there. I told them things had gotten out of hand, and I had borrowed the money."

"And?"

"Richard, I did not know if they would press charges. My friend's dad, our old boss, looked me in the eye and said the coolest thing. He said, 'Well, you owned forty percent of the company, so you only owe us sixty percent of what you took.'"

Larry was spared a legal ordeal. This emboldened him and solidified his trust in God. "I trusted these communications from God more and more." Larry now was taking his driving directions from the Lord. Literally. "I would drive around, taking turns and really not knowing where I would end up."

He is careful to explain that he never heard a voice in his head. He would silently ask questions of the Lord and suddenly just know the answer. Yet he remained mum with everyone except Kimi. "This was not all right to share with people," Larry said. "Instinctively, I knew that. I kept the experiences to myself."

If Larry was losing it, he did so with common sense. "This is hard for people to grasp," he said. "Even in my psychosis, there were islands of reality. Instinctively, I knew there are actions that can increase the possibility of being locked up." He had acquired survival skills. "I had gained those insights. I was no fool."

Discretion prevailed until, at last, enthusiasm overtook him. Kimi had been working desperately to protect him from friends and family, but could not hold him back. "When it all got stronger and more intense, I could not stay silent. I shared my experiences with the rest of my family."

Larry's older half-brother, Bill, found Larry's revelations difficult to take. He had moved away from his own religion and was bothered by Larry's zealotry. "I was put off by Larry's excessive religiosity because of my own rebellion against the Southern Baptists, the dipped-in-the-blood-of-Christ sort of stuff, to the point where it was almost like fingernails on the blackboard to me."

On a summer Sunday afternoon years later, we sat in Bill's comfortable Atlanta home, a far cry from Larry's mountain cabin. Bill's wife, Sally, jumped in. "Bill's friend was a psychiatrist. We consulted him, and he informed us about the nature of mental illness."

"What did he tell you?"

"He made it clear that Larry was very sick."

The family tried to persuade Larry to seek help. He refused. Soon his life began to crumble around him. "During this period, Kimi left me. She was trying to hang on to her life and needed a separation." Kimi had stood by Larry, supportive, even strong. The foundation, though, had cracked. "I frightened her," Larry said. Kimi had been swallowed up by events, overwhelmed by Larry's intense relationship with the Lord. "I was still drinking, and by this time, Kimi had quit. I fully understand she had to leave."

But at that time, Larry's psychosis sent other signals. "I thought it was part of the religious persecution that any apostle of Christ could expect. I was not taking any medication yet. That would be part of Satan's plan. Kimi, my family, doctors, they were all part of Satan's plan. They could not understand I was called to live like people such as John the Baptist, totally committed to my mission."

"Which was?" "Back then, my mission simply was to be a prophet of God, to do whatever God communicated to me." There was no room for doubt.

Brother Bill is an attorney and understood that the family needed a strategy. "My brother is smart," Larry said, chuckling. "He used my relationship with Christ to convince me to seek help. I will never forget him saying, 'Look, you believe this is happening. We love you. Christ is about unconditional love. Out of love for us, would you go into this psychiatric hospital?'"

The answer was instant. "Yes." In 1984, Larry checked into the hospital without resistance. He was placed in a detoxification unit because of his substance abuse. He was now God's warrior in captivity. "God was telling me I had to get out. There was work to do." Six weeks later, having changed his mind about life in the hospital and knowing there was a mission waiting on the outside, he went to court. He had learned a little law from others on the ward and knew his rights. He won his freedom because the hospital stay had been voluntary. Georgia law was clear; no commitment, no confinement.

Larry was not impressed by his diagnosis, manic depression. "These theories were things you have to put up with as a prophet of God." Clearly, the diagnosis meant nothing to him, an attitude that would not change for a long while.

Denial, perhaps? How denial and psychotic behavior combine is anyone's guess. "Denial in psychosis comes when we have our first insight that something may be wrong," Larry said slowly, sounding sure of himself. "We do not want to accept the diagnosis or the prognosis. Then people go off their meds. That can be even worse."

LARRY PROVED NO healthier after his return to freedom, picking up pretty much where he had left off. But now he had an incredible mission. "I was going to fly to South America, to Bogotá, and break up the cocaine cartel." A friend alerted the family, and Larry's father disabled his car to keep the young man close to home.

"This was scary stuff," Larry said. "I was romanticizing law enforcement and the virtues of fighting drug dealers as an instrument of God." He wanted me to understand the manic euphoria he felt. "I would wake up on this dopamine high and want to begin my work each day as a crusader for God. I was fully connected to God."

With Kimi gone, Larry took up residence in a large house, a quadruplex on St. Simon's Island. He had made the purchase with his earnings from the sale of Iceland, renting out three units and keeping one for himself.

St. Simon's Island sits in the Atlantic off the coast of Georgia. As a young network news producer, I had visited refuges there for armadillos and birds.

"This was a beautiful place to be on a manic high," Larry noted. "I would just ride around in my diesel van.

I would pull up next to a police car and smile at the officer driving. I was convinced my car was bugged, and they knew everything I was doing. That was okay," Larry assured me. "This was just part of the plan to bust the drug dealers. I was euphoric."

Larry knew where federal drug agents trained near the island. He arranged a meeting with two agents and informed them that he had a reliable source in the cartel. The agents were interested. Larry did not tell the feds that God was fingering the drug dealers. He simply told them about a bowling alley where deals were going down. The agents seemed to believe him.

"What happened?" I asked.

"I do not have a clue," he admitted.

His half-brother Bill does. Unbeknownst to Larry, Bill had quietly entered the picture, ready to do what was necessary to protect his younger brother. "First of all," Bill said, "Larry had a gun. We were scared to death." Bill had contacted the DEA agent and waved a red flag. In the end, Bill had to steal Larry's gun and passport to keep him around and very possibly alive.

Chronic illness was now striking the entire Fricks family. A close family gets sucked into the crisis, whatever the cause. Larry's family stayed in contact, desperately watching over him. "Yes. We love Larry," Bill's wife, Sally, said. "On my first date with Bill, we watched Larry play in a high school football game."

That is how close Larry and Bill were. Sharing the burden of illness becomes less about obligation than about loyalty and love. "But yes, there also is a responsibility,"

Sally told me. "Sometimes you do not want to get involved, but you have to. That is part of our value system." She paused. "You learn. You cannot close your mind."

Bill and Sally discovered a highly personal payoff that seemed to make the pain worthwhile. "Larry's problems taught us a valuable lesson," Sally pointed out. "One of our kids had a mental health problem involving depression. Drugs and alcohol were part of it," she said quite openly. "Our ability to manage the crisis came from the experiences of living with Larry's problems." She smiled. "This is an illness. Do not freak out."

Unfortunately, the oldest generation of the Fricks family had done just that. Larry's and Bill's parents could neither grasp the scope of the illness nor cope with it. In addition to Larry's increasing psychiatric battles, another son, Stephen, was dying of AIDS. The parents were on overload.

"We are talking about two brothers who were confronted from a social standpoint with two of the most stigmatized experiences you could ask for," Bill pointed out. "Homosexuality and AIDS." Bill paused, looking at his feet. "And then mental illness. Our parents could not deal with either. To be hit with both of those at the same time," Bill continued, shaking his head. "How do you explain the phenomena of all that was happening, especially to religious older folks?"

By the mid-eighties, that battle was in full force. Larry was drinking again, between short bouts of sobriety. "I would set out without money, and God would provide. I once traded a bottle of Vidalia onion salad dressing for a meal." Every successful act of survival reinforced Larry's belief that he was traveling a righteous road.

If he had no money in his pocket, there were funds in the bank. He decided he would invest in the shrimp business off the Georgia coast. "At this time, the shrimp industry was really struggling," he recounted, "but if God is going to show you where the shrimp are, you know, I would have done just great."

"And you believed that."

"When you are in that state of mind, you do not make sound business decisions," he said with a laugh.

And then there was the parrot. Larry had purchased a fifteen-hundred-dollar parrot from a local pet store. "Money means nothing to a person in a manic state. And God intended me to have that bird," Larry explained with a wry smile. "The owner warned me that this was the meanest parrot you ever met. I could not be stopped." Larry bought the bird. "All I remember is Larry driving up in a convertible with that parrot and talking about Jesus," Sally told me.

Larry's actions and attitude grew more irrational and less predictable. Bill and Sally could not summon a smile as they described behavior they were forced to confront. "Larry was running head on, just ramming Coke machines," Sally recounted. "He seemed to go after anything red." Why? "I really do not know," was the subdued reply.

"I can tell you," Larry said casually. "Coca-Cola had cocaine in it, originally. I felt that the Evil Empire of Coca-Cola was founded on cocaine." If he could not take up arms and make it to Bogotá, he would fight the enemy on these shores.

Bill reiterated the frustration the family felt. "Look, we

were not uneducated or totally clueless. We had the ability to call on resources," he said in a strained voice. "But I cannot emphasize enough the pure terror we felt. Here is somebody you love, that you see doing this stuff that is unfathomable, and you cannot change the behavior, which is spinning out of control."

"These must be tough memories."

"Of course, but they are not always clear. On a certain level, you try to block these things out."

Kimi ventured back, unwilling to abandon her husband of little more than a year. Throughout the siege and through the strain, there was something binding, holding them together. The two loved each other. "I did not want a divorce," Larry said. "I had grown up in that southern Baptist culture, where you do anything you can to avoid divorce." But Larry only increased his consumption, using alcohol to hit the brakes on his blossoming mania. "Our relationship was fragile," Larry remembered. Something was going to give.

Larry was careening his way toward a second hospitalization, though he was too well oiled to see it coming. An overwhelmed Kimi got him into the car one night and drove him to the hospital. "I was so drunk, out of control, I have no memory of it," Larry said. Large pieces of his life were evaporating into a drunken fog.

Larry was anything but steady on his feet when he hit the hospital. He collided with the admitting physician as he veered his way into the facility. The chair near the door seemed to flip over backward, and the doctor went flying, tearing his suit in the tumble. The exact details of what happened are not important. What matters is that the institution labeled the mishap a physical attack by a patient. This justified Draconian measures. For as long as Larry was inside, he would be maintained on Thorazine. Larry's voice grew grim just talking about the drug. Bad? "Thorazine is a chemical straitjacket," he said with steel in his voice.

"The drug is a hammer." The pain in Larry's words was clear. "When they put me on the megadose of that drug, I could hardly walk or talk. I remember trying to make it to the nurse's station. Not a chance." He was immobilized. "The mind sends signals, but nothing happens."

Larry continued to stagger his way through the hospitalization, failing or simply refusing to accept that he suffered from a mental illness. Doctors had become the enemy. The view from deep inside the walls of the psychiatric institution instructed that doctors and patients did not play for the same team. "There were psychiatrists who truly believed that recovery is not possible, that we would never be moved through and out of the system."

Finally, Larry had demanded a Christian psychiatrist. "He took me seriously," Larry recalled. "This guy cared." After being released, Larry told the psychiatrist he wanted to take responsibility for his life, to assume ownership of his illness. "This doctor listened and tailored my outpatient treatment to fit my beliefs. He knew I was a serious Christian."

"This guy was feeding you Thorazine, Larry."

"That's true," he responded immediately. "It is true." But, Larry added, his doctor was the one to wean him off the hated drug as well. This psychiatrist did seem to believe in hope.

A drug-assisted assumption of hopelessness makes the patient's job almost impossible. "It is very hard," Larry said. "Doctors who have the hubris to assume a collection of symptoms shuts down the human spirit ought not to be practicing medicine."

No doctor can predict the power of the human spirit. Too often, physicians do not look up from their charts long enough to understand. "Richard, I was exposed to doctors whose eternal hopelessness was all they offered."

Larry was saved by his insurance company. Equitable discovered that Larry had lied on his application about abusing substances and cancelled his policy. He was discharged soon enough. "I honestly believe that the hospitalization was shortened when that money dried up." No surprise there.

FOR A WHILE, Larry functioned normally on the outside. "I came out of the hospital more stable," he says. "I was on my best behavior, sending the right signals to people, and watched how I acted pretty carefully. I was smart about my life at that point." He still believed he had been touched by God, but he observed great discretion in public.

In a last-ditch effort to breathe life into their marriage, Kimi whisked Larry away to the Caribbean. She may also have sensed the nascent depression lurking in him. The two ran from reality to a yoga retreat on Paradise Island in the Bahamas, where Larry followed the rules, for a while.

Then one night, he swung over to the depression side of his illness, riding the bipolar continuum down. If Kimi's Caribbean mission had been to help Larry find peace, his own goal became a secret search for something more lasting.

"I wanted to die," he said. "I was out there, over my head in this beautiful water, trying to figure out how to drown." Even as he sought that final solace in the depths, he failed to complete his objective.

When the couple returned to Georgia, Kimi left Larry for good. Their marriage had lasted just over a year.

"Did she know that as she was ending the marriage, you were trying to end your life?"

"Hell, no," Larry answered. "Kimi was just scared." A trust officer at the bank, a man she long knew, had warned her that any kids they had could carry Larry's illness. "Kimi needed a life," Larry explained. "The time had come."

Larry's feelings of responsibility for what his psychological state brought on his former wife cuts through him to this day. "I hurt that woman badly," the man said. Guilt and shame are common emotions during recovery from mental ailments, Larry explained, measuring his words about the emotional carnage. "I have profoundly strong regrets." He knows his actions were not premeditated, that he could not help himself. He acknowledges that Kimi stood by him until she could not take his behavior anymore.

"Kimi really, really tried very hard to help me. I do not want to create any more pain for her than I already have. I feel very bad about the strain on Kimi and my family." In our years of conversation, Larry could not express his remorse enough. Emotional fallout from illness settles in layers.

WITH THE DEMISE of his marriage, Larry's attention turned to mere survival. He desperately sought work, looking for jobs, anything, but with no success. "I even applied for a job at a local McDonald's." He stopped for a moment. More than money was at stake.

"Richard, I learned that work is so important."

"Tell me more."

"Work for us is treatment. The mentally ill are the most unemployed of any disease group, with an eighty-five percent unemployment rate." The statistics are convincing. These studies indicate that, with the right support, mentally ill workers experience a lasting reduction of symptoms when they are employed.

Strain and pain were reaching a crescendo in Larry's mind. He was alone at the lake house. Kimi had moved out, and Larry had been on his own since their return from the Caribbean. Over a period of weeks, a terrible depression descended on him. He was decimated.

"I got down on my knees and prayed," he recounted quietly. "I was in so much pain." I could see that pain in his eyes as he spoke. "I badly needed relief." He paused for a few moments. I listened to his breathing.

"It gave me peace that I could control something."

"But you were so out of control."

"No." Larry looked straight into my eyes. "I was going to kill myself. That is control." He was calm and quiet as he spoke. "I was going to take an entire bottle of Thorazine I had tucked away from an old prescription. I had the bottle of Thorazine tilted up," he said. "Pills had begun to pour out. Richard, my mouth was open and I was going there." What happened? "The phone rang. It sounds crazy, but the ringing was sudden and very loud," he said. The jarring, almost explosive ring startled him. "Literally, I spit out pills."

The suicide spell was broken. Depression dissipated as mania reappeared over the following weeks. Larry was all over the emotional map, exhibiting erratic, uncontrolled behavior. "That just shows how unpredictable the disease is," he said. In his head and through his body, he was speeding.

"I would sleep for two or three hours and wake up and feel like I could do anything. It was superhuman. I felt absolute clarity and energy, perfect direction."

"But you had just tried to kill yourself," I pointed out.

"Yes, but I was back on the roller coaster, and what I had done did not matter." Larry stopped. "Besides, I was drinking again," he remembered, shaking his head. The pattern was all too clear. Here was a man who badly needed to find the brakes.

Holed up at the Lake Lanier house, Larry was losing touch rapidly. By his own reckoning, he was coming close to a psychotic break. One afternoon, a few days into this siege, he was in the house, drinking heavily. "I remember just sitting around, thinking this is an evil place, satanic. This was where our marriage had fallen apart."

Suddenly, he picked up his keys and walked to the van parked by the house on the water. "I got in, threw the van into drive, floored it, and crashed the thing into the house." Larry recounted the event calmly. "The attack on the house was an attack on all that had gone wrong."

Then he got out of his van and walked away. He did not turn back, even look over his shoulder, as he began a new leg of this strange journey.

Delusions were running the show. "I was convinced that there were children buried in a landfill in Cummings," a nearby town. "A serial killer had placed them there, and God wanted me to go get the serial killer and find the children." So Larry set off on foot, wearing a pair of sweatpants, no shirt, and no shoes.

He came upon a Presbyterian church. "I had come to believe that churches were a diversion from the true teachings of Christ," he said, ever a committed soldier of the God Squad. "I got into a football crouch and attacked the sign in front of the church and knocked it down."

Don Quixote approached the lake. Rather than going around the water, he elected to swim straight across. He dove in, wearing his raggedy uniform, oblivious to the fact that he had left his Speedo at home. "My sweatpants quickly became waterlogged, and the next thing I knew, they were off. I was buck naked."

Larry completed his swim across the lake and found a house. "I knocked, and when a lady answered the door and found this naked man facing her, she started screaming." Larry chortled. "I knew something was wrong. Even when you're psychotic, there are islands of reality within that psychosis. I knew I had crossed a line."

He ran next door to a small weekend cabin that was empty on this weekday afternoon. He broke a glass pane next to the front door and reached in to unlock it. He slipped inside and made himself at home. "God is good, I thought. The owner drank the same wine I drank. His clothes fit me. I took a shower, toweled off, put on his clothes, and sat there in his chair, drinking the guy's wine."

Larry heard a male voice shouting for him to come outside. He walked from the house. The man pointed a rifle at Larry, instructing him to stay there, perfectly still, until the police came. "'Well, you will just have to shoot me,'" Larry remembered saying back to him. "I was thinking I was invincible. Thank God he didn't shoot me. I walked up the driveway, and there was the county deputy waiting."

"I broke the law," said Larry, and noted that he had become a statistic. As government cuts social services, he explained, more and more mentally disturbed people are ending up in jail.

"Criminalization of people with mental illness is reaching epidemic proportions. The Los Angeles jail is the largest psychiatric facility in the country." And chronic mental illness patients all too often become chronic prisoners. This is especially true for minorities and the poor.

"If I had not been white and middle class, I would have been booked, charged, put into jail, and then, what happens to you in jail, especially if you are in a manic state?" Larry said. "This becomes a downward cycle, a trap for the mentally ill."

But Larry's real estate buddy Jim was waiting up the driveway for him, standing with the deputy. "The deputy said he was there to assist me, and I needed to go with him," Larry recalled. "I said, 'Sure.' I got in the deputy's car, and we rode over to the jail. He put me in a cell alone."

Over the years, prisoners had covered the walls with graffiti. Larry began decoding the messy markings, convinced they were messages from the Lord. "God was helping me connect certain letters in a code that no one else would be able to see. I was on a divine mission."

Neither physicians nor family found the mission lofty.

A psychiatrist evaluated Larry and reached the obvious conclusion that he had, in fact, suffered a psychotic break and needed to be hospitalized again.

LARRY HAD RUN out of choices. He was committed by the state, heading for his third hospital stay. The staff was waiting. "When I got out of the car, they sort of jumped me and carried me inside. Jim was still with me, and I remember turning to him and calling him Judas." In Larry's mind, Jim had betrayed God and his servant.

The staff put Larry into a treatment regimen, each time taking him to the same small room. "They forced drugs on me. The doctors can do whatever they want, because the patient is cornered." Larry described his treatment as dehumanizing. "I was in what they called seclusion," he remembered. "People could look in at me through a small opening in the door." He was kept in restraints, bound to the bed.

What Larry cannot recall is what drugs they forced on him or how long he stayed in solitary. The pharmaceutical fog was too thick. "I have no idea what they were putting in me," he said. "It probably was Thorazine." A coldness creeps into Larry's voice as he discusses his care.

Larry found saint and savior among the devils in this forced hospitalization. Each time he entered or left the facility, another patient who also suffered from bipolar illness extended a hand, each time saying the same thing. "'I feel a sense of spirituality and a direct connection with God,' he would say. 'That is real and cannot be taken from me.'"

For Larry, who was starving for human connection,

these fleeting moments had power. "This man was the first person I saw who understood me. He did not say, 'Oh, that is all psychotic. Your awakening is not real.' This man just said, 'Look, I believe you.'"

Years later, Larry wrote in the *The Journal of Dual Diagnosis* about the power of meeting that individual. "My trusted peer had walked in my shoes and was not confronting my spiritual journey . . . as a psychological disorder." Writing the experiences of illness had become an important piece of Larry's own recovery, a way for him to establish perspective.

Too often, he said, what happens in forced treatment is that medical people act without thinking. Doctors force patients into non-psychotic behavior with such zealotry that they dismiss too many possibly positive and healthy dimensions of the patient's mind and soul. They do not tolerate eccentricity or unconventional views.

Sometimes a fine line separates psychosis and off-center belief. According to Larry, conventional wisdom is not the only game in town. "In casting those judgments," he said to me, "they dismiss what is your reality."

Larry crawled out of that institution a broken man. The lake house was on the market, and Larry's parents had stored his belongings in their basement. Proceeds of the lake house sale were to go to Kimi. "That was the least I could do for her." Larry paused and went one step further. "I was crushed by this sense of the absolute hopelessness of my life." He seemed to be giving up.

During one drunken evening out, a call for help from Larry's date brought his father to the scene. Larry says he was sick of interference from others and in a confrontational moment with his dad, Larry tackled him to the ground. Then he drove away.

Larry and I sat on his porch on Buzzard Mountain as his story reached its denouement. The faint sounds of leaves rustling in the breeze made Atlanta seem far away. Larry told me about one powerful moment, a single act so long ago. "I buried my wallet," he told me. "Larry Fricks could be no more." This was twenty years ago, but he remembers clearly the meaning of that act.

"Everybody wanted me to go back to being who I had been at one time," he told me. He defined that as a crazy John Belushi character. "That guy had crashed and burned long ago." Memory of the moment, the night a life came unglued and an identity vanished, was powerful.

Larry purchased a six-pack of beer and checked into a Holiday Inn the night he wrestled with his father. Larry had run out of fuel. Nothing of the man remained. "I lay on the floor. I cried, 'God, help me change,'" he recalled. "I fell into the fetal position, and I cried again. I felt such shame. Where had I sunk to?"

"I called my father later that night. 'Okay,' he said. 'I will pick you up,' adding, 'No, we are not going to put you back in the hospital.'"

Larry had crossed a wide river during those predawn hours. The excesses of Buckhead were far away. He says he made a pact with God that night. He would continue to believe in his spiritual awakening, though he knew the rest of his life would have to change. "I knew that the way I was going, I would end up in and out of psychiatric hospitals for the rest of my life," he said. "I needed new people and places and things." This beleaguered man set out on a new leg of his journey.

PAIN AND SUFFERING, the ordeal of so many years, had forged a new sensibility. "I chose not to be angry or to give up," Larry says with the conviction of a convert. "To be transformed would be to live to my potential. Recovery would mean a transformation for me, to realize I could own my life. I knew I had to take action."

Larry began to repay debts. He got rid of the new RV, which had been purchased on credit. He sold all his properties. And he stopped drinking.

More tools than determination would become necessary to put this troubled soul on track. "I was disabled," he recalled. "I would just sit in the morning, staring at the closet. I could not decide what to put on. I could not read a book. My concentration was gone." Still, he was determined not to fall back on old patterns.

He volunteered to work with elderly patients at a nursing home, which became valuable therapy for him. Just as Buzz looked to the dying to teach him how to live, Larry turned to lonely, disconnected old folks to slip back into society. He concedes that he identified with their desperation. "The lives of these people appeared more hopeless than mine. I worked with them and got outside of myself."

Larry accepted medication, and began taking lithium. "I had pushed medication away for a long time, which was a big part of the problem." He struggled with the side effects of the medication. "I had shot up to three hundred pounds by now because of the lithium." He started to lift weights under the tutelage of a new friend, Paul, who was a former Olympic weightlifter.

Although the pain was still all around him, he knew he could not play victim but had to become part of the solution. "I took responsibility," he told me emphatically, a phrase he would repeat many times. That act meant learning and dealing with the realities of his disease. "I realized just how bad sleep deprivation is. I learned I can control my sleep patterns with medication even when I awaken in the middle of the night."

Self-awareness led to proactive involvement in his own care. Eating nutritionally balanced meals became important for Larry in maintaining the chemical balance in his body. "The diet thing was kind of tough," he said. "I had to just make myself do it." His spirit, though, remained in tatters.

"I was in desperate need of a sense of purpose." I was putting out résumés, searching for jobs everywhere. This was a long way from my career as the general manager of an ice skating rink."

"Were you honest about your past?"

"I could not bring myself to tell the whole truth," he admitted. "There were holes in the résumés. I could not explain where I had been."

"Did you feel guilty about that?"

"What you should say about the past is a question I never stop asking."

Larry was contacted by his former real-estate partner Glen. "He invited me to live with him in his condo and proposed a new real-estate partnership." The pair formed a new company and bought a sixty-acre property. It was a good move for Larry in more than one way. The land had a house on it, and Larry moved in. "It was in Lumpkin County, which was dry," he noted. When the property eventually sold, Larry stayed in Lumpkin.

"I also wanted to be of service and realized that real estate was not the way to do that," he continued. "I began working with kids. They were troubled children, juveniles with alcohol and drug problems." And Larry renewed his passion for journalism and began to write again. "Writing gave me something meaningful to do with my life during the day. I would use writing to get an identity back. I sent my columns to local papers."

Larry hit a small gusher. "One local editor liked my work and encouraged me. He started publishing my stuff." Seeing success was empowering. "I would see my byline and begin to weep," he said, his voice cracking. "I realized I could make a contribution."

"Did you make a living writing?"

"Hell, Richard, I made twenty-five dollars a column."

Fledgling success had a seismic impact on him though. "It was a very important part of my recovery."

"How so?"

"It meant that I had meaning and a reason to get up every day."

"Did you see yourself as damaged goods?"

"There is a real trauma factor that other illnesses do not have. If you are sick and a pain in the ass to your wife, there is no danger of doctors taking you away to forced treatment."

Journalists need boundless self-confidence to put themselves on the line, the hubris to stand by their stories and insist they are right. "Oh, yeah," Larry said in a low voice. "I had a fear that if any story was wrong in any way, there would be consequences."

"You mean your past."

"Someone would go right to my illness. Always, I was looking over my shoulder."

"Were you a tough critic?"

"I demanded exacting standards of writing for myself every day. I think I had to work harder than anybody else just to satisfy myself. I did not want to compromise my credibility. I built a network of people I trusted and who trusted me, and that worked."

Those of us who fight illness battle on two fronts. We fight both the disease and public ignorance. That survival mechanism minimizes new wounds but does not hide the scars. Larry needed a more personal connection.

"I WAS ALONE because I was not worthy of another person. I really did believe that." Larry's lithium weight gain only accented his loneliness. "That was one reason I became even more reclusive, at least until Grace came along."

Larry's wife Grace was working as an advocate for the developmentally disabled in Georgia when they met. "I was just as much drawn to her life values as to the fact this was a beautiful woman," Larry explained. "You have to connect on the big issues. In the end, that is more important than anything else."

Grace offered the same sentiment. "It is the values that keep people together." Then she began to laugh again. "Hey, wait a minute," she shouted. "We are regular people, you know. We like food. A lot. We love the outdoors, our dogs. A lot. And Larry is very funny."

What Grace was speaking to is a curious misconception about any couple living with a chronic illness. Folks seem to believe that illness dominates dinner conversation. "They think the illness is the center of everything," Grace observed, "but it is not." You mean there is more to life than being crazy? "Look, Richard, we talk about policy issues or workshops or books we have read on the general subject, not Larry's specific illness. We also talk about movies and art and what we read in the paper this morning." I totally understood. It's not as if Meredith and I sit around talking about degeneration of the central nervous system!

The frustration in Grace's voice was evident. "What people believe about mental illness and about someone sick can be worse than the disease itself." That statement echoes from Larry as well. "I was put in this diagnostic box and could not get out. If I get excited about anything, people say, 'No, that is a symptom of your illness.' If I get upset, 'No, this is your illness.'" Larry's emotion now was apparent. "When does the diagnosis stop and the human being regain a sense of control of a life?"

I WAS IN a taxi headed for a generic motor lodge on the outskirts of New Haven where I was going to watch Larry work. Even though I knew him well and felt comfortable in his presence, I felt slightly ill at ease.

This morning, I would sit surrounded by individuals, real people, who suffered from debilitating mental illnesses. This would be a field trip for me to watch and listen. Larry would be running training sessions, teaching the seriously sick to help one another and, of course, themselves.

The cab pulled off the busy highway and onto an access road as trucks and buses and assorted maniacal motorists screamed by. Soon we were in the parking lot of the least charming place I could imagine. An alienating locale seemed an ironic venue for a gathering of the mentally challenged.

Larry had explained that he and his colleagues believed the mentally ill would listen to one who had walked in their shoes. "They want to hear from each other," Larry said, "people who have been there and understand. Not some doctor who does not get it." Larry preaches self-reliance.

I fumbled to pay the driver from the wad of loose singles in my pocket. There was Larry, stout and smiling, standing in wait at the door. We headed for the basement. Participants gradually moved into the windowless conference room. They arrived in clusters. These were regular folks, chatting away, certainly appearing animated. People kept coming in, even as Larry began to speak.

I sat silently, staring and studying appearances and mannerisms. Men and women smiled, going out of their way to be welcoming, even to sit with me. They shook hands and offered more coffee. Many carried pad and paper, and as we broke into small groups, they laid the materials across the tables before them. They were serious about what they were there to accomplish. Many seemed to know one another and were easy with Larry. That comfort derived, quite plainly, from his comfort with them.

"These are people who have lost faith in the world,"

Larry told me later. "They are searching for a new connection, struggling to find that faith again." He thought for a moment. "That is hard work."

WATCHING LARRY AND GRACE at their cabin-like home in the mountains becomes an exercise in mutual comfort: synchronicity, to be exact. Harmony in the house begins early in the morning, with gourmet coffee delivered to the bedroom by Larry. The man adores his wife.

"I do not know if you are aware of this, but Grace once took over a state psychiatric hospital that was in receivership," Larry said. "She turned it around with toughness and extraordinary empathy. She really is tough, brilliant and tough."

Grace also suffers from clinical depression. "I do not know if that is part of our connection," she said. "I am grateful that it does not bother Larry."

"But look at his history."

"Yes, but when you are depressed, it is a downer for everyone around. Even when someone understands, you get tired of it."

Grace was not on antidepressants or any such medication when she met Larry. "I was worried about stigma," she explained. "Always. I did not want any evidence around. Larry convinced me to do something about the depression." He told her she is great. "He kept telling me he loves the total package."

"Do you think you are mentally ill?"

"Maybe," Grace answered. "I never thought of that. I guess clinical depression is a mental illness."

"Are you both better people for that?"

"Without depression, maybe we would not be as empathetic. Maybe we are nicer."

Larry weighed in. "Grace never experienced the psychosis that takes away your soul. She never had to undergo forced treatment." Obviously, that becomes its own category, but the stigma applies to anyone who is mentally ill. "Grace does not buy into this stuff that life is over when you are ill." Larry put up his hand. "Grace just rolls her eyes when people say the mentally ill cannot live in the community."

With most people, it would seem fair to ask if there were qualms marrying someone with a mental illness. "No," said Grace in response to that question. "We are soul mates. Our lives do not center on Larry's mental illness but his mission to de-stigmatize it." Larry nodded. "When we started going out," he added, "Grace was less concerned about my mental illness than I was."

Grace seems unyieldingly proud of their lives, who they are, what they battle. "Richard, let me try to explain something," she started. "There are a lot of high-profile people in Georgia who have different mental illnesses. So many people know us and Larry's work. They are encouraged, helped in their lives." Grace was emotional. "Mental illness to us is a badge of honor."

Grace and Larry are childless, though not because of concerns about genetic possibilities. "It just happened that way," Grace said. "I was thirty-eight when we got married. We figured, if it happens, it was meant to happen." But there seem to be no concerns about passing the illness down. "Not at all," Grace agreed.

Chronic illness is all about managing. Larry stays away

from alcohol because he must, although he watched Grace drink wine with me in their living room with some interest.

"Is it tempting?" I asked.

"Not really," he answered, "but occasionally I see someone drinking Scotch, and I have to say, it looks good."

"Do you feel victimized?"

"Not at all," he answered quickly. "Grace would not let me internalize my issues or become a victim." Larry smiled. "I am not sure there is a better person in the world for me than Grace."

Grace is tuned in to Larry. She becomes his muse, taking in his ideas and reacting. "I get excited and get all these ideas. I bounce off of her." Grace appreciates that role. "We have a great time," she said. She watches for any warning signals of Larry losing his footing. "I can tell when Larry gets overly anxious or is overtired or working too hard."

"I had lost the belief in myself," says Larry. "Grace helped me find that again."

THAT BELIEF IN self shifted in 1990 when Larry spontaneously went public about his past. The impact of that moment turned him from journalist to advocate. "I was attending a commissioners' meeting to discuss a community program. The plan was like daycare for mentally ill people."

Opposition to the project from the local citizenry was strong. "There was a not-in-my-backyard quality to the debate," Larry said. "People said things that were very discriminatory." He sighed. "The whole thing was insulting, I thought."

"Given your own history, you must have felt weird," I said.

"I was upset and did something very unprofessional," Larry said quietly. "I told the people there that I was in recovery from a mental illness. I said I had been hospitalized and that the stigma is unbelievable. We have to give these people a chance," he told the commissioners. "Well, you could have heard a pin drop. They gulped, and then they passed the proposal."

And an advocate was born.

Larry had been to hell and back and now his spirit soared. "Religion is for people who fear hell," Larry told me. "Spirituality is for those who have been there." Life to Larry is not about a church but belief in the human spirit. "Richard, that spirit is why I get up each day." For him, doctors did not understand this dimension.

"Psychiatry tried to beat it out of me, to convince me this was just a symptom of my disease, a psychiatric disorder."

"And that was not the whole story?"

"No. Spirituality is different from religion. Even in sickness, I see a spiritual realm that to me is real." Religion was gone from Larry's life, replaced by a spiritual sense that tells him to reach out to others.

So Larry was ready for the phone call he received from a state mental health director. Would Larry attend a statewide meeting to set up a mental health consumer network? Larry accepted and became the volunteer coordinator. He and his new colleagues began work on the organization. Larry kept his newspaper day job to underwrite this volunteer work.

His words that afternoon at the meeting in the mountains and his move toward advocacy made a private and highly personal process public. "The term 'recovery' is fairly recent in mental health," Larry observed. "I had to think hard about whether or not I wanted to deal with the publicity, the pain that would go with it." He went silent. "I had been there already."

Of course, he could have stayed silent at the advocacy proposal. "I could not break away from the calling," he said, "but I did not answer them about their job offer for a few days." He weighed the consequences. "I wrestled with it. I was doing well as a journalist. I could not imagine the passion this would unlock. But nothing I ever have done has motivated me more."

In addition to setting up a mental health consumer network, Larry volunteered to find a location for a mental health conference. Proprietors quickly backed off when they leaned that conference participants would include those recently out of recovery from mental illness.

Larry's pent-up anger had a new utility. He aimed it at an ignorant world and at the psychiatric establishment. The imprecision of those doctors, he says, throws human beings into diagnostic containers that may not fit.

"They told me my life was hopeless," he said, "that I would never get it back. The medical establishment thinks it has the right to take away hope, based on a diagnosis that is, at best, confusing." The medical profession acts with paternalism, he says, playing an inappropriate role that does not necessarily serve the sick. "I get very angry at this," he admitted.

And I thought *I* was the archbishop of anger. Years of MS and cancer had unraveled me more than occasionally.

Larry, to his credit, emotes for others. But while my anger can be combustion for its own sake, Larry's is channeled, generating electricity, which, of course, is power.

"I still have a reservoir of anger that I have to live with," Larry said.

"Is anyone listening?"

"I do not know," he answered. "You know, we are dangerous," he paused, then went on. "They have to silence the insane, the mentally ill, because we tell the truth."

"I know people who had jobs and may not have revealed they had a mental illness," Larry said. "If and when they had a relapse and went into the hospital, when they came back, the job was gone."

"Living with any chronic illness can get you screwed at work," I said.

"Well, there is a big debate in the mental health community, to disclose or not to disclose." And? "Under the Americans with Disabilities Act, you do not have to say anything."

I told Larry I vote for self-protection. He nodded. "No one is immune from discrimination," he answered. "One of the great stories is about the president of the Georgia Mental Health Consumer Network." What happened? "He went in to renew his driver's license. There was a form that asked, 'Have you ever been treated for a mental illness?' If you checked 'Yes,' they pull you out of line. They also ask about medication. Talk about profiling." He laughed.

If there is an American prejudice against all people suffering sickness, a special stigma does seem reserved for those who battle diseases of the mind. "The common portrayal of an individual with a mental condition is of a violent person," Larry said. When a bomb exploded at the Atlanta Olympics in 1996, early newspaper accounts attributed the incident to a crazy person. "The headline always reads, 'Mentally ill man beats wife.' You don't see that with MS." Fair enough.

In 1999, during the final years of the Clinton administration, Larry spoke to a White House conference where the first surgeon general's report on mental health was being released. During the meeting, Larry introduced Tipper Gore and spoke of the genetic component in his family's war with diseases of the mind.

"As a child, I used to sit with my grandmother as she stared at the fire warming her living room," Larry told the conference. "She would rock and stare, and sometimes an impish smile would creep across her face. I loved her deep, infectious laugh. After giving birth to her youngest child, she experienced mental illness. For all the years that I knew her, no one ever talked about her psychiatric hospitalization, or why she never ventured beyond the fence surrounding her home."

That Larry had made the journey from the wild experience of mental illness to the White House was lost on no one in the Fricks family. His brother Bill silently wept as Larry spoke.

"What I really regret is that both parents died well before Larry's recovery." Bill looked away. "To be recognized at the White House for what you have accomplished . . ." he trailed off. "All they knew was the pain." Bill had to pause. "Bless their hearts, both of them. They did not see him come out the other side."

Before Larry's White House talk ended, he described

the price he paid for his moments of madness. "Never had I imagined that one day I would be four-cornered in the bed of a psychiatric hospital, having people stare at me through a small window in the door." And then he talked about a place that haunts him to this day.

"When I was a high school senior in Atlanta," he told the conference attendees, "we took a field trip to Milledgeville. Up to thirty thousand people have been buried on the hospital grounds. We walked through wards and gawked at the patients. I remember feeling ashamed to be intruding on these outcasts of society."

ARE YOU A man of hope? "Hope is to the soul what oxygen is to the body," he answered. It was a Saturday night and Larry was heading, once again, to the Atlanta airport, this time flying off to a mental health conference in Australia. "This will be your last shot at me, buddy," he had warned me over his cell phone, which, of course, was fading in and out. "Make it good."

As I thought for a moment, Larry kept talking. "Hope to me is the key to recovery. We can encourage hope with practices every day." How? "I start each day reading something hopeful. I really do."

"You have lost a lot in your life."

"Let me tell you, I would change nothing." That gave me pause. "If you tried to take away my illness, if you could make it just disappear, I would say, 'No. No.'"

"Strong stuff, Larry."

"To take my illness," Larry continued, "would be to remove the meaning and purpose I now have. Mine is a purposeful life."

"Your illness has overtaken your identity."

"I was somebody else, a different person before I went through this."

MILLEDGEVILLE HAD FELT lonely on that September day when Larry and I visited. I remember seeing a marker by the restored gates to the cemetery. An elderly gentleman suffering from bipolar disorder had raised the funds needed to commemorate the spot. He had no known link to the place, no horror stories connected to the facility. And when he died, it had been by his own hand.

A lone figure can be seen in the distance among the graves. It is a bronze angel that Larry and other advocates, all sufferers of mental illness, had donated to Milledgeville. The figure stands as a memorial to the nameless, faceless victims buried all around.

"They may have been powerless in their lives," Larry observed, "but the message of what they experienced has come through from beyond the grave." The angel stands in silence. One arm extends up to the heavens, the other hangs limp toward the ground. The circuit is complete.

....

Reflections

Dueling with Ignorance

Preparing to meet Larry, I became uncomfortably aware that I had a dark image of this mentally ill man. Yet when

I finally came face-to-face with him, there were no signs of instability, no signal of a psychiatric condition. Quirks or crazy talk were not to be seen or heard. That stereotype of this stranger was decidedly wrong. Larry was just a guy.

My concerns had been only half-serious, but that 50 percent bothered me. My private thoughts clearly revealed a troubling discomfort with a disability many of us know little about but view as threatening. So while Larry is your average fully functional adult, he has to prove his normalcy to the world every day. His challenge is to deal with us. There stands the extra hurdle in an already difficult life.

I wear my own illnesses on my sleeve and speak openly about my experience of illness. Larry's psychiatric disorder is buried deep in his head. For years it has stayed hidden, a secret sickness locked away from an unkind world. Since public ignorance breeds stigma, an indigestible staple of Larry's diet, Larry long ago had to learn the serious business of self-protection.

We should know better than to automatically anticipate the worst when we engage a person with a mental disorder, perhaps I in particular. Nearly a decade ago, my physical reaction to morphine after cancer surgery brought hallucinations and frightening psychotic behavior. That brief window onto a mind unleashed brought me close, albeit briefly, to the experience of mental illness. Few events in my life have left me more shaken. Where was my empathy for Larry? Perhaps I was expecting to meet a man out of whack because I had felt like one when my opiate receptors went mad.

Larry reminds us all that a picture-perfect façade may not be a reflection of an impeccable interior. Appearances may be half-truths at best. We all have hidden frailties and weaknesses. But add a mental illness to the mix and a caricature in the minds of many is born. Those among us with mental disorders are judged.

My initial fear of Larry was unfair. People can write off the mentally ill with cruel indifference. Yet so many of our problems stand small next to Larry's. A broken leg mends, but a mental illness only can be controlled. And so we watch the mentally ill and wait for the eruption we assume will come. We place them in a cold room in our minds.

What has been taken from any victim of crushing illness will not be returned. For Larry, the pain of public stigma only adds weight to his shoulders. Larry must travel one step at a time, battling his condition and the closed minds around him.

seven

Coming Together

OUR MINI-MOTORCADE MADE its way across Boston, moving slowly down Longwood Avenue toward the main quadrangle of the Harvard Medical School. No pomp or pageantry carried us, only a handful of taxis and one disability van equipped for a wheelchair.

Everyone was a bit nervous. Moving from home to Harvard had been a leap of faith. The five principals had met for the first time for dinner at the Harvard Club only the night before. Together we broke bread and plenty of ice. And the dialogue began. The meal had been a rehearsal. The big show waited across town.

Our entourage had splintered almost as quickly as it formed this afternoon. Cars and cabs, buses and assorted commercial vehicles, roaring through Boston's old streets had cut into the group and carved it up, leaving us in pieces.

What was left of our caravan drove past hospitals and labs and slowed as we approached the medical school complex. The place was impressive, looking very much like the separate city it is.

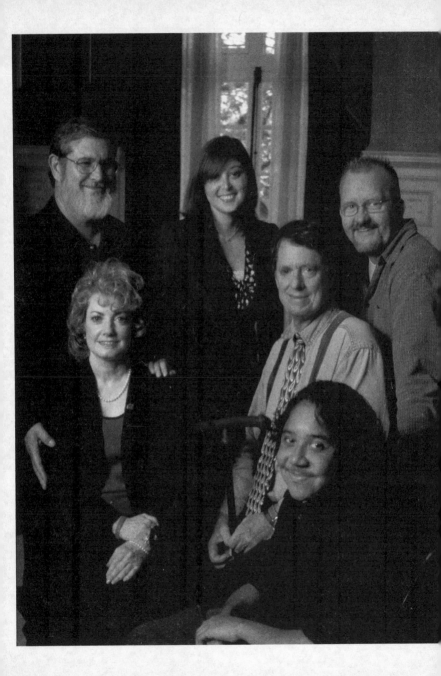

I had wished that we would all cross the main quadrangle together on foot. The setting was stirring, but walking was out of the question for Denise and Ben. Stones and steps and mere distance put the trek out of reach for me, too.

We had spent the morning gathered around a grand table at the Harvard Club. With rolling audiotape our only witness, we shared experiences with an intimacy and candor that seemed unusual for relative strangers. Crumbling health provides a powerful common denominator for individuals whose only connection is sickness.

Now we were going to share our difficult lives with the next generation of doctors. Medical students, with faculty and guests in attendance, would bear witness to five individuals with chronic illnesses swallowing hard and revealing themselves. Such exposition was new at Harvard, we were told, which was news to me.

We entered a back door and, in short order, walked into the well of a large amphitheater that was more vertical than horizontal. For all I knew, this might have been where autopsies once were performed in this mysterious institution. Or was that only in old movies? Perhaps this was an apt metaphor for individuals preparing to put private parts of their lives on the table and into public view.

A young medical student read portions of the preface to *Strong at the Broken Places*. "These are faces of illness in America," she intoned. "Do not look away." The five participants sat straight and nodded, looking at one another and hearing those words for the first time.

They stared in anticipation. Their families sat on stools in a narrow space behind. All spoke of the hurdles before them, openly, sometimes emotionally. These five individuals were playing to a packed house. And they were there for the right reasons.

These unassuming folks—folks is exactly who they were—had arrived in Boston in search of something very different: community. Solidarity derives from connecting with others traveling the same road. Instinctively each recognized that their chorus produced power beyond any solo. These folks were at Harvard now, and they were in charge.

As always, their stories were authentic. I felt so proud of them.

"Sarah," I began, "a long time ago you described yourself to me as 'defective.' I know how much you meant that, but you have always looked to others to define normalcy."

"Who knows what normal is?" she interrupted. "I look at my peers, my friends, and I feel like I am less of a person than they are because of this disease that I carry with me every day. I do feel defective."

"You are a successful woman, but still that is how you see yourself?"

"I see myself as, I guess, not a whole me. I am not a whole person." Silence sounded. Sarah became animated. "I have to defend myself, and I am sort of a broken person."

"But defend yourself against whom?"

"The world," she answered.

Buzz nodded. "Yes, it is the world. Everyone looks for perfection. You are supposed to be this way or that, and then it turns out, you are not." He looked across the audience. "You are ill. There are days that I cannot get up.

There are days I just feel like crap. Yet I have got to go on. I've got to prove to them I am going to do this. I am going to get up, and I am going to walk forward and not look backward."

"Is that about proving something to others or proving it to yourself?"

"For me it is both. You know, I am not going to let this defeat me. I am going to defeat it."

"Is there a goal in that?"

"Yeah," Buzz answered. "Every day is a goal. Every day I wake up is a positive. It is good for me."

"People do not get that, do they?"

"No," Buzz answered instantly. "No one is supposed to be ill. I mean, in the perfect society there would be no illness. But here we are."

"Don't people accept that?"

Buzz scoffed. "We have friends who do not come around us because I guess they are fearful of getting it. I say, 'You cannot catch it. This is not something you catch.'"

Ben spoke up. "I want initially to prove things to others and to myself. I have to go through every day saying, okay, how am I going to do this? Am I going to be negative? Am I going to be mean to people? Because, in fact, most people I come into contact with are nice."

"I believe there are dimensions to chronic illness that are just miserable," I offered. "There is nothing sexy about chronic illness. Women die of cancer with great flair on the silver screen all the time. But the slow suffering of chronic illness is the anti-Hollywood. Even if it's treatable, it just plods along, unresolved, incurable. It rules our lives. Does anybody relate to the idea that we just become our illness?"

"Yes. I do," Denise yelled out in her slurred voice. "Of course, ALS has totally changed my life. I was diagnosed in the last five years, and it is all that I do, everything I think about. I take a step. Do not fall on your face. What am I going to eat? Oh, it has to be soft with gravy. How am I going to get in a car? Who is driving? How can I go to the market?" At this point, Denise had to pause just to breathe. "This is everyday life," she wheezed.

"This is the hidden daily burden of sickness," I told the audience. "It is the small stuff that gets you. What doctor asks about that?"

"I will have days when I say having this disability really sucks," Ben said suddenly. "But I guess I really have not resolved my feelings."

"Are you resigned to a limited life, to accepting all the things you cannot do?"

"There are always going to be moments where you're like, why am I even here?" Ben seemed focused. "Why am I even bothering to try? But that is just setting yourself up for failure, screwing yourself up. I think no matter how bad your condition, that even the smallest element of a positive attitude can get you through things."

"Do you agree with that?" I asked Denise.

"Oh, yeah," she said in that breathy voice of hers. "Even just a little bit of hope or a moment of fun can make me happy. I believe in fun, and being happy. And having purpose keeps me going."

"Do doctors understand the therapeutic value of those things?"

"Some understand."

"Is it important for a doctor to understand?"

"Hell, yeah, it matters. That person is a better doctor for understanding how the patient feels."

"Sometimes you have to put your own sickness away," I said. "Ben, I used to go for days without remembering that I have multiple sclerosis. Do you ever forget that you live with muscular dystrophy?"

"I would have to say, I am consistently aware of it," he responded. "There is not a minute or even a second that goes by." He paused. "Well, probably a couple of seconds, but I guess there is always a moment every part of your day where you think, okay, I know I am not normal. Then you just go on with your day."

"So you left for college and moved away from the security of everything you had grown up with. How did you feel about dealing with new people?"

"I became introverted because I was scared," Ben answered. "Basically, I did not know how other people would perceive me."

"What were your fears?"

"Here I am, young, black. In a wheelchair. I am like, okay, there is a double whammy in terms of minority status. Not only am I African American, but I am also in a wheelchair, and I am trying to balance those two out. How am I going to cope with being a double minority in this college setting, away from home, without the familiar support systems I am used to? I am going to have to forge and create new ones."

"Fears surrounding how others are going to see you must be powerful, especially for young people. Sarah, your years of treatment with powerful steroids for Crohn's took a toll on you, physically and emotionally."

"When I say I feel like a defective person, it's because my whole GI tract is defective and not normal and because of the side effects from taking steroids."

"Which are?"

"I have a round face," Sarah said unemotionally. "Sometimes I feel I am defined by my looks. I always wonder if other people notice or think to themselves, why is her face so round? She is a very small, petite person. Every time I look in the mirror, that's the only thing I see, is my round face."

"All of us can see a caricature of ourselves staring out from the mirror. That cartoon character is manufactured in our heads, isn't it?"

"Except that society buys into that view of us without resistance," Larry said, referring to mental illness, "and then we own it."

"True. Sarah, you look like you are ready to explode."

"That has always been an issue for me. When I was younger, people used to say to my parents, 'Oh, my gosh, what is wrong with her? What is wrong with her face?'"

"Was that just when you were little?"

"No. Throughout high school I would have people look at me and make comments, not knowing what a touchy subject it was. So that definitely, with my physical appearance, has been a huge thing for me. Having the added stress of the physical side effects of medication is that every day, every second, I am reminded that I am defective."

"Denise, do you agree with Sarah and Ben, that the world sees you as a caricature of yourself?"

"Absolutely. It is true. People have misconceptions," Denise said clearly. "We upset the apple cart by being ill.

This cannot be reality. People do not know how to deal with us. Who is asking them to deal with anything?" she asked rhetorically.

"Larry, correct me if I'm wrong, but your mental illness probably provides the greatest opportunity for people to caricature illness. It must be like whiplash. You struggle to know who you are and to feel good about yourself. At the same time, people are coming at you like you are from a science fiction movie."

"Yes, but there are good things that come out of the experiences, too."

"What?"

"I think we have a greater opportunity for transformation when we have dealt with something life-changing like living with a mental or any other serious illness." He gestured to his right. "A great example is Ben," he said, turning to look at the young man. "Last night, I went into the restroom, and realized you could not have used that restroom." All eyes turned to Ben. "Yeah," was all Ben said, slowly nodding.

"Before I had my illness," Larry continued, "and before I began to grasp how people with disability are treated, I would not have had that insight or that awareness. But my feeling is, you know, I ain't goin' anywhere Ben cannot go." Larry wore resolve on his face. "I ain't goin' anywhere Ben can't go," he repeated for emphasis. "I feel the same about the rest of you. I just don't know you as well. I talked to Ben about a lot of this stuff last night. We are linked on that."

"Larry, you look for the good in any bad situation."

"When you have these experiences, you start to realize

that diversity is actually very much a growing experience, and hanging out with people who have had these experiences has created some of the greatest moments of my life. I would not give back those moments."

"But moments are not always so great, are they?"

"I have a lot of positives in my life," Sarah conceded, "but it is inevitable that, for me at least, I am going to have times where I say, 'This just really sucks. Woe is me. What good is there in my life? I am this defective person. Who is going to want me? Who is going to want to marry me? I am a burden on my family, on my friends.' It brings you down." (Sarah could not know her life would change a year later and she would have her answers.)

"Of course," I halfway interrupted, "you know that none of that is true."

"Yes." Sarah laughed. "I do."

"But that does not matter, right?"

"It does not." Sarah paused. "As I have said before, I have become a self-deprecating person."

"This is common among the sick because, somehow, we decide the disease is our fault."

"Yes," agreed Sarah. "Sometimes it is hard for me to accept that these things are not true."

"Denise, can you describe how the reactions of others to your evident disability have hurt you? You said you wanted to look sensational for this meeting and seminar. How does that fit in?"

"Absolutely. I did," she exclaimed. "People do not look at me as a female anymore. They see me as a woman on a walker, someone with a terrible disability."

"You mean, the disability is all they can see?"

"Right. That is the beginning and the end," she said. "And why would they want to get involved with someone who is so sick, especially when there are so many healthy people."

"Should they give it a chance with you?"

"Why bother?" she answered curtly. "I am dying." Denise was abrupt. She continued. "They see the walker and wonder how old I am. Then I speak, and then they are very curious as to just what I have been drinking. Then they *really* look at you, like, 'Oh, my gosh. She's already had the best years of her life.'" In a healthy world, we can be written off very quickly.

I was struck by the silence in the amphitheater. Faculty and students were moved by the obvious strength of the participants.

"I constantly feel like a burden to everyone," Sarah said to the assembly. Illness conflates with guilt, especially in the young. "I am always apologizing to my friends if I have to cancel plans or end a night early, whatever, because I just feel run down. That is one thing that I am always apologizing for with my peers and people that I work with. With my family, I have this tremendous feeling of guilt that since age four, I have been this huge burden to them."

Joan, Sarah's mom, objected strongly. "I have never for one day or one moment thought, I wish I had a child who was perfect, because I know young women, and there is none who is perfect. They all are flawed. Girls have difficulties, and I think girls especially are hard to raise. But Sarah was no harder to raise than a girl in good health. Sarah is a normal young woman."

"But, Joan, we have talked about your relationship with

Sarah, which is a close relationship and greatly affected by her illness."

"That is true. From the moment of Sarah's diagnosis, I was a very controlling parent."

"Was that just because you are that kind of person, or was it the medical circumstances or both?"

"I think that the circumstances demanded control, and my husband is a very articulate, very bright person, but he falls apart in a medical situation. He is not able to cope. So somebody had to cope, and that was going to be me. So in that way, I kind of felt I had to take control."

"The biggest control issue for me," Ben said, "was making the transition from walking to being in a chair permanently. That was basically a big step for all of us."

"Ben, why do you think your folks pushed for the chair?"

"My parents did not want me to collapse anymore. But I was reluctant, I guess, to use this power chair."

"Why?"

"Because there are certain stigmas associated with people who use power chairs. I was neglecting to control myself," said Ben, looking up and out at the students. "My parents were trying to teach that to me, saying, 'Listen, you have an ability to go out on your own and do your own stuff. You talk about control. Well, actually, practice what you preach.'"

"Control is a powerful issue with sickness, isn't it?"

"For me, as a man, it is large," Buzz said. "For patients I deal with at hospice, it is the same thing."

"Meaning?"

"We do not feel useful in our family's life." What about

losing control over your own body? "Losing that control is just awful," Buzz added. "I was constantly throwing up. I had no control. That was the worst experience."

"How did it make you feel?"

"I felt defeated. I could not control my bodily functions."

I wonder if doctors understand the psychological burden of losing control, and if they would care if they did understand. A physician once told me that he wants to provide the best science he can, making clear that he has little interest in holding a patient's hand.

"Do doctors understand that when absolute control is gone, the struggle to hold on to some form of power can mean so much to the sick? Even our own families may not get it."

"Oh, yes," Buzz quickly responded. "This is what my family copes with, twenty-four/seven."

"Buzz, does Susan get it?"

"No. Not always. She cannot know." Buzz stopped. "People are different. They cannot always understand everything. When I am working at the hospice, I never say, 'I know how you feel,' because I do not know. Imagine the loss of control there. Nobody really understands, and I do not expect Susan to. She cannot."

A man in the audience took the microphone to address family members directly.

"I think it was Buzz who said that it's not your disease. It is your family's disease. Could you talk about to what extent that is a common theme, and how you approach it?"

Sarah's mother, Joan, spoke first. "Since Sarah has been ill for most of her life, we really do not know what it would have been like to raise a child who was not ill." Her voice tightened. "I think that you have to make it your mission, and you have to be your child's advocate every step of the way." She continued, "We were given words of advice early on by a pediatric gastroenterologist, who said, 'You can take this child home and make her an invalid, or you can take this child home and make her everything she can be.' That was really the guiding principle of Sarah's life."

Debi, Ben's mother, took the microphone from Joan. "I have to echo what she just said. Ben was diagnosed with muscular dystrophy at three, and we got all the facts and figures, and what to expect. My husband and I sat, and we talked, and we made a decision. It was going to be all about quality of life for Ben."

"Meaning?"

"We made a conscious decision that he was going to have a normal life. We were not going to coddle him, because in our minds, he was going to grow up to be a young man. He was going to go into manhood, and he had to have the skill sets that he would need to function."

"Do you guys think of yourselves as strong people? To others listening and looking at you, you do project strength. Ben?"

"To some degree, yes," he responded thoughtfully. "I guess I'm more of a humble person than that. I do not want to brag too much about things."

"You can be strong and humble, Ben. John Wayne pulled it off."

"Well, I am not John Wayne by any stretch of the imagination," he said, flashing a broad smile. "Yeah," he added. "Elements of strength separate me from others. But at the same time, I think everybody may have a particular situation that is tough for them but easy for others, whether we are disabled or not. It is not only about disability. I believe that everybody's strength is relative. It is what they make of it."

"Buzz, has cancer made you strong?"

"Stronger," he corrected me. "I have learned to be stronger. I have learned to take charge. Instead of cancer defeating me, I'm going to defeat the cancer. That is the attitude I have to take. We have run across . . ." Buzz looked up into the seats above. "How many of you are studying to be doctors?" A multitude of hands went up. "Okay, this is what a doctor should not do. I will tell you this flat out. I was extremely, extremely ill. I had driven myself to the hospital, crawled into the cancer center, and crawled up to the desk. The woman there could not even see me. She just thought this voice was talking to her. But I was on the floor." He started to describe what happened next, but backed off, asking his wife, Susan, to pick up the story.

"I work in the ER," Susan began, "and they called me and said that Buzz was really sick. In a matter of minutes, I got there, and Buzz and I started talking about what might be going on and about our son. I started crying. The doctor came in and said, 'This is nothing to cry over.' When I get mad, I cry more, so I cried even harder. And he said, 'Like I said before, this is nothing to cry over.'" The look on Susan's face as she told her story said it all.

"I wanted to say, 'You do not even know me,'" Susan said in a shaky voice. "I did not say that. I did say something to one of the nurses, and she said 'You need to tell the administrator of the cancer center.' Later, this doctor came back groveling, and he said, 'If you need anything over the weekend, you let me know.'"

Susan looked up. "Buzz, as sick as he was, lifted his head, turned, and said, 'You would be the last one we would call.'" Buzz smiled at his Harvard audience. "There was a time when I never would have said that."

A woman in the amphitheater spoke up. "This is a question for Buzz, Sarah, and Larry. I was wondering if you feel you have faced any additional difficulties with your illnesses that to the outside world are not visible?"

Sarah began. "A great example of that is my first job out of graduate school as a social worker. I was going through weekly transfusions and iron infusions. I lost my job. Obviously they did not say that my Crohn's and all the side effects were why I lost the job, but I was missing a lot of work. It was obvious." Sarah continued. "Because of the steroids, my face was full, my cheeks red. I looked healthy. People just think, oh, she gets stomachaches a lot. Go take some Tylenol. That is not how it works."

"We fight our illnesses," I said, "and we do battle with so many of the people in our lives. The indifference of others, coupled with the stigma that people attach to physical imperfection, doubles the difficulty of living with illness. Larry, I have to believe that of the illnesses represented around this table, mental illness is stigmatized most. Maybe in our history of discrimination, there is little difference between the M word and the N word."

"There might be some disagreement there," Larry responded. "I will say that there is no illness except maybe leprosy where patients are lifted up and removed from the community." He pointed out that as he grew up, his church prayed for the sick but not the mentally ill. "We suffer in silence."

"I have not walked in anybody else's shoes," he said, gesturing to the others in the amphitheater as well, "or been in their wheelchairs, so I cannot really speak for them. But I would suppose that what adds to the stigma of those of us in recovery from mental illness is the element of forced treatment."

"Being committed," I said, "and locked up."

"I don't think anyone else here would ride to the hospital in the back of a police car. That is kind of a disempowering experience, when you are in the back of that police car and you yell to your neighbors, 'Hey, I got to get to the hospital. Feed the dog. Don't know when I'll be back.'"

I glanced around. Everyone was staring silently at Larry. "There is the fact that we are still segregating people in institutions," he continued. "I mean, it's not over yet, folks. We have people in those institutions in Georgia that have been there almost all their lives."

"If there is a common thread binding these five, it is their dissatisfaction with the doctors in their lives. Do you think that the stigma attached to mental illness is made worse by doctors?"

"I think the good docs would even acknowledge that." Larry answered.

"Oh, yeah," Buzz agreed. "I understand what Larry is saying. The doctors do not live it every day the way we do. As far as some of them are concerned, you are your stigma. You know, with Denise or Ben, you see the devastation. Mental illness is in the shadows, maybe where cancer was twenty years ago. Doctors set the tone."

"I had internalized the hopelessness," Larry told the group. "If you were to ask a group of clinicians what disables people with psychiatric illness the most, they would say the symptoms. If you ask us, most of us will say it's the stigma of the disease and the poor self-image that results. That is more disabling." Symptoms can be controlled by drugs and therapy. Stigma runs rampant in the minds of others.

"I do believe that doctors bear some responsibility for creating the attitudes that we all bring to chronic illness. Buzz had told me long ago that he had been stuck with one doctor who could not look him in the eye because of his admitted discomfort."

Larry's wife, Grace, took the idea of discomfort to a new level for the medical students. "As the spouse of a person with mental illness, I have to say that many times people who know that Larry has bipolar will turn to me to answer questions for him or act as if he is not even in the room." Grace spoke carefully to the students. "So, as a spouse, I have to learn how to step back so that the person himself, in this case my husband, is pushed forward and speaks for himself."

I jumped in with a similar experience. "My wife and I went to a religious service, and she was parking the car. I walked into the back, and the usher stared at me. She did not come over. She saw the cane. She kept staring at me. I stared back. My wife came in, and the woman immediately walked over and asked, '"Where would he like to sit?"' The murmuring told me the audience got it.

"This stuff happens," I continued. "This is not just

about mental illness. It tells us how other people see all of the sick. I was at Amtrak in Washington, waiting to get on a train. An agent came over to prepare and open the gate. She said into her walkie-talkie, '"I have three canes here. I am going to board the canes first.' So I started to hand her my cane." Uncomfortable laughter sounded around the amphitheater.

"We are objectified, and these kinds of experiences become daily occurrences in our lives. And we all know it. Eventually we become accustomed to the insensitivity of others. Gradually, we think less of ourselves, and expect rejection. Ben, how do you respond to that?"

"I have realized that a lot of that stigma was inside of my head, that I imagine the worst thing possible as absolutely occurring." He was talking about female friendships. "In fact, there are plenty of young women who are some of my close friends in college, whom I talk to a lot, eat with and hang out with."

"And what have you learned?"

"I realized that basically it was up to me to actually put myself out there, to discover what people are really about, which is that I think most people are inherently good."

"That took a while, didn't it?"

"It did."

"Did you get help?"

"Yeah, but you got to do it yourself."

Larry pointed a finger at our group to make a point about stigma. "Last night at dinner, people made comments about insanity and it was humorous, but is that something everybody should laugh about?" He was looking at me.

"Larry, you use humor and make jokes yourself to make people comfortable with you."

"Absolutely," Larry responded. "What I worry about," he continued, "is what I call the soft discrimination of low expectations. I was a journalist. I owned a business once, but I am often confronted by people who expect nothing from me. I think I am fortunate that there are times when I am just doing really well, and have learned to manage it." It can be tough to demand of yourself when others expect so little.

Then came a question that each of the five chose to address. "To what extent did you seek out or were you sought out for support by different social groups or nonprofits that deal with your disease, and what, if any, were those experiences like for you?"

Ben spoke up first. "My parents said, 'Okay, we are going to try and do something about this and be as proactive as possible.' I am real fortunate to be able to work with folks from the Muscular Dystrophy Association. MDA has been there time and time again. I am more than satisfied and very grateful."

"Denise, more than once, you said to me, 'I was an unhappy person before I got ALS, and that changed.' On the face of it, that sounds, well, weird."

Denise giggled. "When I was diagnosed, for about eight months I really did nothing, ended my job, and a friend got me involved with the ALS Association Greater L.A. chapter. I started volunteering and hanging out and writing letters in the quarterly paper, speaking at seminars, at schools. A year and a half ago, I was asked to be a Board Trustee. They are my saviors."

"That changed your identity, didn't it?"

"Yes. Advocacy gave me an identity. I am far more at ease with the disease, because I know what is going to happen. I am an advocate. I see my future, and I live life every day until I cannot move. That is why I went to Antarctica two years ago. Now I could not go. With their help, I keep pushing myself. Last year, I did Paris with a cane, took thirteen trains a day, walked down every step. Now I cannot."

"Buzz, you said you felt used by one advocacy group."

"They just wanted to use me as their poster boy. Then I came to find out that only thirty-three percent of the dollars there go to research. Everything else goes for salaries and such things. Where is the patient in this? Where is the research? Do not showcase someone like me and say, 'This is for research' when it is not. I pulled away and now I am working with the Leukemia and Lymphoma Society."

"I am on the boards of two very good organizations," Larry told the group. "The National Mental Health Association, and the Depression and Bipolar Support Alliance, with more than one thousand support groups across the country. I think they are making a difference."

"I have had an incredibly positive experience with the Crohn's and Colitis Foundation," Sarah chimed in. "When I went away to college, I had an amazing doctor there who was very involved in the CCFA, and hooked me up with the Greater Atlanta Chapter. I was asked to speak in my freshman year, and then I volunteered at a camp that's offered for kids with Crohn's disease and also colitis. I became their poster child. I created a camp in Cleveland for kids with those diseases. I have had a great experience with them."

"I think advocacy for all of us is all about taking ownership and allowing illness in. The terminally healthy may not recognize the significance of that step toward making peace with ourselves. Those of us who have grappled with our demons and the cold world recognize the distance of the leap toward self-acceptance."

A member of the audience provocatively suggested that advocating for changes in the workplace or in public places could be interpreted as the sick asking for handouts. There was silence. "I do not speak for anybody here," I said, "but I do not think that is what we are talking about. Those who suffer from chronic illness are not begging for special consideration. We ask only to be treated with the same respect and similar opportunity as everybody else."

What grabbed everyone's attention was something Denise said about my own long struggle with multiple sclerosis. "I do not want what you have."

"Excuse me? Denise, you have ALS."

She nodded. "You know," Denise continued, "not being able to see and walk around freely." The medical students appeared puzzled.

"Let's go there," I responded.

"Look," she said to me. "I care so much about photography. To not shoot photos would be horrific."

"I get that," I told her. "But you think I am dependent?"

"Yeah. I have spent a lot of time with you. You are so dependent on people. You do not drive anymore. You have trouble crossing the street alone."

"But Denise," I said softly. "You are going to be totally dependent on others for everything."

"I know." She paused. "That is right. I am, and that kills me." I could hear her breathing. "Dependence is worse than dying."

I had observed during our years together that many among us tended to view others as having it worse than they did. I guess we are all more comfortable with the devil we know.

WE LEFT HARVARD Medical School with sobering testimony echoing through our heads. A tribute from the podium gave heart to five individuals who had offered very personal accounts of their struggles with sickness. "I want to say that in fifteen years teaching here now," Dr. David Cardozo told the gathering, "this is the best experience that I have had and the most useful.

"We have learned a tremendous amount from you," he said, turning to the participants. "Hopefully we are going to be better scientists and doctors and human beings after the experience."

Cardozo believes the youngest minds in medicine are open to change. "This will alter the direction of their training. Perhaps young medical minds will take a new shape. I think some will be inspired to work on chronic diseases."

A conquering army, or maybe a guerrilla squad, returned to the Harvard Club for a last meal together. We patients had spoken our minds and the doctors were listening. Maybe we were heard. We celebrated our small victory.

Before going our separate ways, the group planned to tour the historic sights of Boston. Buzz and Susan's son, Ryan, had shown up in Boston clutching a history book and a wish list of historic sights to visit that he had drawn up with Grandma's assistance. Ryan had seemed oblivious to our agenda, no doubt by intent. During our sessions at the Harvard Club, he had wandered away from illness, heading over to a wall of watercolors of Bunker Hill and other Revolutionary War scenes.

We took the tour. And then we were gone.

"We are in touch by e-mail," Buzz told me only days later. The group had carried their dialogue home. I was eager to know more.

Of the participants, he said, "They were great. There were no attitudes." And what did Buzz learn? "I was amazed at how the diseases are different, but they have one thing in common." Which is? "People without a voice," he answered. "I get tired of beating my head against a wall because I have no voice. Now I do not feel so alone. The meetings made me stronger and more determined."

"Buzz, did you talk about the trip at church?"

"Oh, yes. They were amazed and said I have more fire now. Someone said my testimony is powerful. Let me tell you. Buzz Bay has a voice now."

"You had it before, Buzz."

"I know," he laughed. "Maybe I hear it better now."

Later, a revealing e-mail from him arrived. "Ryan calls us Richard's Team and you are our coach." I read that as the sad wish of a little boy who hoped someone would save his Dad. Who better than a coach?

Buzz's e-mail continued. "To say who surprised me the

most, it was Sarah. I had envisioned an emaciated individual, but she is a ball of fire, knows what she wants and how to get there."

All seemed to be in awe of one another and energized by their meeting. Sarah was struck by how positive everyone at the Boston event was. "I was amazed at how they approach life." And the medical school audience? "I felt the seminar made an impression on the students." In what way? "I think doctors have preconceived notions about the sick. We really are people. We do have lives. Doctors do need to consider that."

"I believe that we helped the medical students and ourselves at the same time," Ben told me after he was home. "If they will become better doctors, we learned more about ourselves by talking and sharing our experiences. I took a lot away. Maybe I will grow."

I had contacted Denise to get her take on the Harvard meeting, wanting to know if anyone had made an impression on her. "I have such respect for Sarah. So far my illness is tolerable. With pain and weight problems, bleeding and bowel issues, I would have killed myself. I want a better quality of life than that. I do not know how Sarah does it."

As for Ben, "What he said at the meetings. Wow." I had told Denise in advance that Ben might stay silent. "For someone who does not speak, oh my God. He is a kid of twenty who is an adult of fifty, with a phenomenal philosophy. Ben had to grow up faster than any kid, realizing what he is going to go through. His outlook on life is extraordinary."

Denise said she had strong reactions to Buzz and Larry

in one-on-one conversations at breakfasts or over coffee. "They really hit me. Buzz has a fatal, incurable disease. I felt close to him in that regard. I am not putting down the others, but there is more of a connection with Buzz because he is going to die."

"With Larry," she went on, "I did not realize how much he had been affected by me. I showed him thank-you notes from young kids who talked with me about ALS. Larry was very moved. Also, he and I talked about volunteerism. It was a good give-and-take. Meeting someone new and having an impact right away is a strong experience." And Larry, I pointed out, is someone with his own problems. "Yeah, big time."

Larry did not wait to be asked for his reaction. His enthusiastic e-mail arrived in New York almost as soon as I did. "As I ride around the Appalachian Mountains, I find myself reflecting frequently on the conversations we had in group settings and one-on-one. For example: I have been wearing a red wrist band Denise gave me that says 'Never Give Up,' and on several occasions, that message has transformed how I handled a present situation."

The next line gave me pause. "Denise shared something when we had breakfast together that has stayed with me. And a conversation I had with Buzz entered my thoughts, and both are impacting my life daily." That raised one obvious question: So, what did they say to you? I reached Larry at his mountain office near Atlanta.

"We had this moment in Boston. Five of us were connected for just three days." Larry paused. "Richard," he said, "that is a brief time."

"Yeah," I slowly responded.

"We were a community that came together."

"Yeah?"

"Three days with those five people brought clarity to my thinking. We are connected, and we were strong at the broken places."

Larry was taken with the fresh view of a younger generation. "I miss Ben's insights. I wish I had the perspective Ben has when I was in college. He gives me hope for the world and evolved communities where all are welcome."

"What about Buzz?" I asked. "What was that conversation you had with *him* about?"

"Buzz is a powerful man," Larry said. "You cannot convince me that his thoughts about life and his faith have had no impact on his body. I believe Buzz has that much power over the cells in his body."

"I do not know about that kind of power, Larry. Maybe."

"The cancer has stopped dead in its tracks."

"For now," I said.

"Yeah. For now, but I believe that is no accident."

"And what about that conversation with Denise?"

"Let me tell you about something that happened," Larry said, barely suppressing a laugh. "We were sitting at the Harvard Club. Denise was drinking water. Her glass had a speck in it." Larry paused, then described Denise sticking her finger into the glass and flicking the speck away. "'It is not like that is going to kill me,' she said." I could hear the emotion in Larry's voice. "Richard, we both started laughing." The meaning of the anecdote was escaping me.

"I cannot tell you what a moment this was for my soul. It was so uplifting for me."

"Why, Larry?"

"Because we were living in the moment. What we have is right now, magnified by momentary insight. Does that make sense, Richard?" I was not certain. "I cannot stand chronically normal people," Larry added. "I love people who appreciate life. They are more inspiring."

"Certainly," I added, "they are more interesting."

"Richard," Larry said abruptly. "Did you know that Denise has a pistol?"

Silence echoed through my head as the computer search automatically began. Did I know? "I am not sure," I answered, which sounded implausible, even to me. Yet the stray fact of a gun did sound familiar. "I almost did not tell you," Larry said.

Faint memory, perhaps disconnected by discomfort, suggested Denise may have told me that as a woman living alone, she needed a weapon. Larry had a different take. "Denise does not think anyone understands her profound depression. Having the gun seems to make her feel she is in control." Control is such a looming issue for Denise.

"Why did she tell you?"

"I do not know. She just told me she has a .38."

Years of conversation with Denise about drawing lines and deciding how far to allow the ALS to progress suggest that she is keeping her options open. Suddenly the subject seemed different. Maybe Denise does have a plan. I was not sure what to do with that thought and decided to think about it for a while. I was in no hurry to confront Denise about actions and choices I respected. Still, I wanted to know.

Denise was in New York with friends a month after we

left Harvard. Christmas was fast approaching. I told her what Larry had said about the pistol. She melted.

"This was a very difficult year," she said very slowly, clearly taken aback. "I have been very depressed, having to go on the walker and giving up traveling. I may have visited my last exotic destination."

"But the gun, Denise, what about the gun?"

"I do not know," she said haltingly, her voice growing soft and trailing off. She seemed surprisingly to be without words. "I think I am over it."

"Denise, would you ever use that pistol?"

"I doubt it." She stopped for a moment. "There are other ways, more peaceful ways, if that moment comes."

I had found an essay written by Catherine Royce called, "I Always Have a Choice." Royce is an ALS patient who writes about living with the disease.

"Every day I choose not only how I will live, but *if* I will live." I heard the echo of Denise's voice in Royce's words. "I have no particular religious mandate that forbids contemplating a shorter life, an action that would deny this disease its ultimate expression. But this is where my belief in choice truly finds its power. I can choose to see ALS as nothing more than a death sentence, or I can choose to see it as an invitation—an opportunity to learn who I truly am."

ON OUR LAST night together in Boston, the group had presented me with a faux Harvard gift certificate entitling RMC "to enroll in one semester of Anger Management 101 to combat his rage." To my astonishment, anger did not rank high in the inventory of emotions carted around by my new friends. Anger has always been too useful a coping mechanism for me to abandon. Yet no one seemed to have the time to be angry, except me. Still, I was ready to matriculate. Maybe my anger could be muted by the new life lessons of others.

"The subject we have not talked about is the power of today," Larry had said, hushing the group that evening. "That is my spirituality, the power of today. Even having to hang out with a guy like Richard, I mean, that is okay. I guess." Almost everyone had laughed.

"We have to let go of yesterday," he continued. "There is not a whole lot I can do about tomorrow. But man, this moment, hanging out with these four people and you and the families. That is real life. That is right now. And this is the stage we are on." Buzz jumped in. "You've got to live in that moment."

Larry hit it back. "You've got that right." There was quiet. "I could be dead tomorrow," Buzz added. "I mean, all of us could. Anything could happen. But now, you take what you have and live."

"Do you feel like you live in the moment?" I asked.

"I have had to learn to do that. I live for what is happening at this time," Buzz answered. "I had yesterday. I got through it. Will I wake up tomorrow? I do not know. I do not know that."

"This is a function of shifting the way you live because of your illness," I suggested.

"Or personal transformation," Larry responded. "That is right," Buzz said quickly. "Because I do not think my faith was as strong until I got cancer." That could have gone either way, I suggested. "I think my faith has really solidified because I had to depend on something much higher than me to get me through this. Doctors were not doing it. They gave up. They said there was nothing more they can do; you are basically on your own."

"You can never anticipate how high the human spirit can soar," Larry added. "I mean, the people in this room are defying what the docs have said. And I would believe that common to all of us is that we depend heavily on a thing called hope. It is a form of faith. It sustains me daily."

Our bottom line in Boston had been hope. The idea is not new but ever elusive for those who are suffering. Said Ben's mother, Debi, "When Ben was diagnosed, what my husband and I were not given was hope. The doctor had none to share."

"When did hope come?"

"Hope came slowly from talking to each other and with other parents. Hope also came from all the emotions we shared over the years."

Hope is as difficult to maintain as it is to find. "When I see Ben, even as he is getting weaker, he is not giving into it. That helps me. He has matured so much, and he keeps going."

"Does that make life more bearable for you?"

"I get my hope through him. Ben's spirit keeps me going."

Debi pushes her son to keep going. "I look at him and say, Ben, this is not all about you. It is bigger than you." Debi sounded so controlled. "Each of us is put on this earth with a purpose."

Adding a final thought, Debi said, "Maybe your purpose is that others can see strength in you. I said to Ben, 'Get over it. Pick yourself up and be positive. You have a lot to offer this world. Have faith.'"

We had left Harvard for a less rarified world and the routine grind of our struggles. My hope, I had told the folks around the table, is peace for those who face and fear uncertain futures. We battle illnesses and fight fiercely but we all need to remain productive members of our worlds.

We can only hope the indifferent around us, next door and down the block or around the corner, will view us as more than our diagnoses and find value in who we are and what we can offer.

I HAD REACHED out to others to witness their battles and in the end become better at fighting my own. I had learned that we each approach the mysterious task of coping a little differently, but we constantly search for answers. The thing about the sick is that we think about these issues because we have to.

We aspire to live and have good lives, defining exactly what that means as we go along, all the while dealing with an ever-changing physical landscape. We all want to live normally and function in the community. We certainly do not want special treatment; indeed, we want to be the same as everyone else.

We withdraw resilience from our emotional banks a bit at a time, praying we are not overdrawing our accounts. We are stronger than we know. Perhaps that assertion is more hope than certainty because we so need it to be. Believing provides the fuel we need to keep going even when we doubt ourselves or believe we never will make it through the day, let alone the night.

I awaken each day and hate being a sick person. But dealing with disability has become a calling. And after writing this book and learning from the gentle people who trusted me and themselves enough to embark on this journey, I now understand that we sick travel together. In spirit, we are one.

And on that day when we cannot walk and words can come no more, we will stand together. When we no longer break bread with one another, still we will sit at the same table. Our hearts will stay strong. In thought and with spirit, we will fly. Our own compasses point the way, and the winds forever will be at our backs.

Please Share Your Stories

ONE OF THE most important things I learned while writing this book is the power of telling and sharing our stories. The struggles of life with chronic illness are numerous and different for everyone, and I want to know about your struggles, your highs and lows, and the joys and setbacks of dealing with sickness while trying to lead a normal life.

I would also like to hear from those of you who are caregivers, you who are so often ignored as you carry the special burden of caring for others while living your own lives. I intend to post many of these stories on the *Strong at the Broken Places* website for all to share in and gain strength.

We, the sick, are a community. We need a place to gather. The *Strong at the Broken Places* website, *www.strongatthebrokenplaces.com*, will serve as such a meeting place. We will be posting regular updates on Denise, Buzz, Ben, Sarah, and Larry. You will be able to find links to information about chronic illnesses. And you can take part in the message board, where any topic is up for discussion.

You are not alone in your illness; you are not alone in your experiences with the trials of chronic illness. I hope you will visit the website *www.strongatthebrokenplaces.com* to share your stories and read about the lives of others.

ALSO BY RICHARD M. COHEN

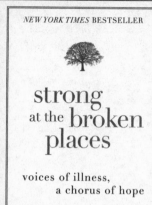

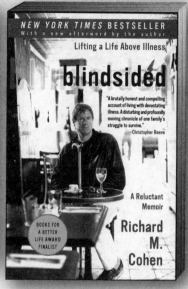

STRONG AT THE BROKEN PLACES
Voices of Illness, a Chorus of Hope

ISBN 978-0-06-076312-1 (paperback)

An honest and inspirational reflection on chronic illness, chronicling a year in the lives of five individuals with incurable diseases.

"The strength of these profiles derives from Cohen's focus on chronic illnesses that, as he notes, are not 'sexy' and generally 'do not resolve themselves'.... These are stories dense with quotidian details."

—*Washington Post*

BLINDSIDED
Lifting a Life Above Illness

ISBN 978-0-06-001410-0 (paperback)

"*Blindsided* is a powerful memoir, tough in the way Cohen's old news bosses would have wanted to be tough. It doesn't flinch and it doesn't whine."

—*New York Times Book Review*

"This is the rare 'illness book' that never swerves into self-pity and never turns preachy; Cohen instead chooses a human mixture of bitterness, anger, and grace." —*Chicago Tribune*